A book by Flax Guru

Awesome Flax

Miraculous Anti-ageing Divine Food

Disclaimer: The information given in this book is presented for educational purposes only and is not intended to diagnose or prescribe for any medical or psychological condition, nor to prevent, treat, mitigate or cure any disease. This information is not intended to replace a one-on-one relationship with a doctor or qualified healthcare professional, but rather a sharing of knowledge and information based on research and experience.

Dedication

I dedicate this book to you my Dad, you taught me science, literature and everything I need to know.

I dedicate this book to you my darling Usha for your kindness, devotion, and making wonderful flax oil muesli whenever I needed energy. You witnesses every moment of making this book.

I dedicate this book to you my sweet Aishvarya for encouragement and endless support you gave me at every step of making this book.

I am thankful to Dr. Arun Nema who helped me for making corrections, typos and suggestions.

Dr. Om Verma

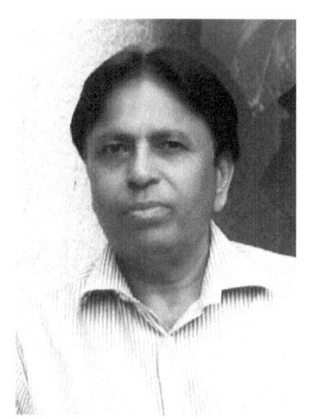

Written by
Dr. Om Verma
M.B.B.S., M.R.S.H. (London)
President,
Flax Awareness Society
7-B-43, Mahaveer Nagar III, Kota (Raj.)
http://flaxindia.blogspot.in
http://budwig.in
+919460816360

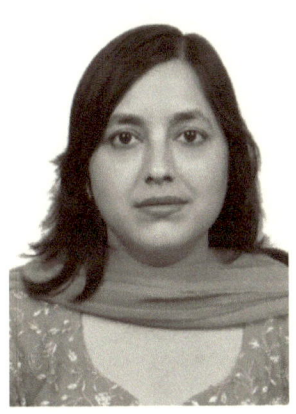

Editor
Aishvarya Sharma
B.Tech Chemical
I.T. B.H.U.
A-304, Raheja Residency, Bangalore

Table of Content

Flaxseed - Miraculous Anti-ageing Divine Food _____*1*

   History _____2

   Ancient Uses of Flaxseeds and Oil _____3

   Making of Flax Oil _____4

   Composition of flaxseed _____6

How Linseed became Flaxseed?? _____7

Devotional Song of Goddess Linseed _____9

Flaxseed – Storehouse of Essential Fats _____14

   Functions of omega-3 _____16

   Cis and Trans configuration _____17

   Prostaglandins - Overview _____19

   Prostaglandins - Functions _____20

   Omega-6 / Omega-3 Metabolic Pathways_____21

   Metabolism of ALA _____25

Lignans - 7 Star Nutrient of the Millennium _____28

   Nectar of Rejuvenation_____29

   Lignans - Elixir of Womanhood_____31

   Heart friendly _____32

   Cancer killer_____33

   Acne _____34

   Baldness_____35

   Protector of manhood _____35

   New hope to AIDS patients _____36

Why should you take a lignan dietary supplement?_____37

*Funda of Fabulous fiber*_____38

Constituents of Dietary Fiber _____38

Soluble fiber _____39

Insoluble fiber _____40

Mucilage _____42

Constipation _____42

Ulcerative Colitis _____43

Journey of Fiber through food canal _____44

*Flaxseed and the Immune System*_____47

Uses of Flaxseed in autoimmune diseases _____49

*Atherosclerosis and Flaxseeds*_____50

Flaxseed protect fatal Arrhythmias _____54

What is diabetes? _____57

Preventing Diabetes by daily Flaxseed consumption _____58

Flax for Diabetes _____58

How to incorporate flax in your diet _____63

Some Natural Remedies for Diabetes _____64

*Science of Memory*_____67

Hippocmpus – The Site for Memory Building _____69

Omega-3 - A Natural Crime Cutter ? _____73

Flaxseed - Sim Card of Mind _____74

*Budwig Protocol*_____77

What is the prime cause of Cancer?_____77

Federal Institute where Dr. Budwig worked _____81

Budwig Protocol _____83

Precautions _____ 92

Prohibitions of Budwig Protocol _____ 94

Eldi oil _____ 96

Coffee Enema _____ 100

Epsom bath _____ 103

Soda bicarb bath _____ 104

Sun Therapy_____ 105

Oleolox – Budwig butter_____ 105

Energy Healing _____ 108

Juicing for the Budwig Protocol _____ 109

Budwig- Compatible Pain Therapies _____ 112

Budwig Diet & Protocol - In Brief_____ 117

Skin _____ 122

Hair _____ 125

Nail – The Barometer of your health _____ 129

Flaxseed and Osteoarthritis _____ 131

*Flax– Good for athletes as well as weight watchers !!!*__ 135

Adding flaxseed to your diet _____ 138

Sprouting flaxseeds _____ 142

Testimonials and Letters _____ 145

Dr. O.P.Tandon _____ 145

Mrs. Dessa_____ 145

Jai Prakash Narayan _____ 145

Dheeraj Sharma _____ 146

Anil Paul_____ 147

Keshavram Bhakt _____ 147

Raman A Patel _____148

Prakash Jain - Flax cured his Arthritis _____149

Achala Kalra_____149

Ravi Kant Prasad _____150

Miss Pooja _____151

Anita Sahai _____151

Flaxseed - Miraculous Anti-ageing Divine Food

What is Flaxseed and how can it benefit me? I was thinking about this question when I started hearing about Flaxseed not very long ago. Flaxseed was a 'buzz word' worldwide and seems to be making great role in increased health for many. I wanted to travel in this wagon of wellness and so I researched until I felt satisfied that it could help me, too. These are my findings.

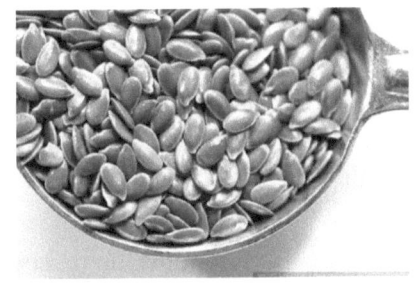

Flaxseeds are slightly larger than sesame seeds and have a hard shell that is smooth and shiny. Their color ranges from deep amber to reddish brown depending upon whether the flax is of the golden or brown variety. The cup-shaped annual, flax flower begins blooming in December and will continue through February, producing abundant blue flowers. Flax may reach two feet or more at maturity. Botanical name of flaxseed is Linum usitatissimum, which has been widely used for thousands of years as a source of food, clothing and decorating houses (paints, varnish, linoleum flooring etc.). Usitatissimum means useful seeds. The plant's common name, flax, is Middle English, originally from the Old English fleax, and related to the German flachs that means to plait, or interweave, such as in braiding.

The crushed seed makes a very useful poultice sometimes in combination with mustard seeds in the treatment of ulceration, abscesses, deep-seated inflammations and even skin cancers.

Flaxseeds have become very popular recently, because they are a richest source of the Omega 3 essential fatty acid; known as Alpha Linolenic Acid (ALA), lignans a phytoestrogen and fiber.

People in the new millennium may see flaxseed as an important new food super star.

Flaxseed increase oxygen consumption at the cellular level resulting in increased energy vitality and stamina and feeling of well-being. In fact, there's nobody who won't benefit by adding flaxseed to his or her diet. It benefits from head to toe and from cradle to grave.

History

Archeological remains indicate that several plants were first cultivated about the same time in Mesopotamia before traveling southward to Egypt. These plants included flax, wheat, barley, peas, lentils and chickpeas.

The Babylonians have been the earliest people to cultivate flax as a food. Linen was used to wrap the mummies of ancient Egypt dating back at least 5,000 BCE. In his epic poem The Iliad (8th century BCE) Homer writes that linen was used for cord and sail-cloth, an indication that the Greeks were cultivating flax plants and were also consuming the seeds. Linen was the fabric used in garments worn by Jewish High Priests. The curtains of the tabernacle were woven of linen.

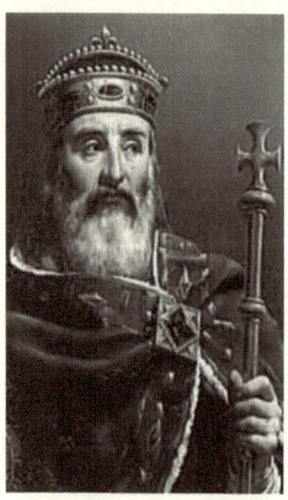

Hippocrates (460 to 377 BCE), a Greek physician who is called the "Father of Medicine," recognized the value of flax in relieving numerous intestinal disorders. When he prescribed flax, his patients benefited from its healing properties.

Charlemagne, the 8th century King of France, regarded flax so highly for its health benefits that he made detailed entries in his medical law books that pertained to the cultivation and use of flax as food and medicine. He ordered

2

his people to consume flax to maintain health and prevent disease.

During the middle Ages, the flax flowers were believed to be a protection against sorcery. The Bohemians, who occupied the area that is now Prague, had a belief that centered on seven-year-old children. Families brought their children to dance among the flax fields because their faith that ritual would make the children beautiful. The ritual also recognized that the entire field was under the protection of a Teuton mythological goddess named Hulda, who is said to have passed on her art of growing, spinning, and weaving the flax to mortals.

Flaxseeds were grown in India for centuries and were consumed as a food grain. Mahatma Gandhi once said, "Whenever flaxseeds become a regular food item among the people, there will be better health."

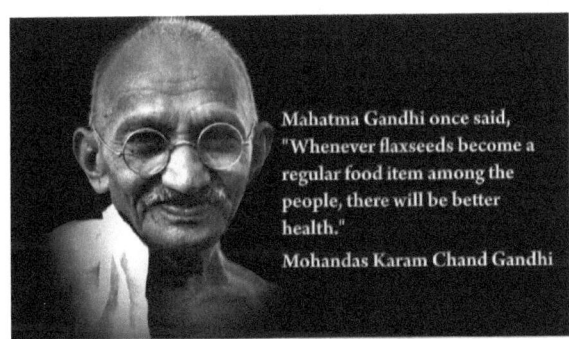

Mahatma Gandhi once said, "Whenever flaxseeds become a regular food item among the people, there will be better health."

Mohandas Karam Chand Gandhi

By the 16th century flax cultivation for linen production was a growing industry that brought wealth to local farmers. During this period flaxseeds were consumed as a common food source throughout Europe. Germans, especially, were incorporating them into a variety of whole-grain breads.

Today, flax is grown in Canada and the northern areas of Europe as an alternative crop. The flaxseed has become popular among health conscious Europeans and are readily available in health food stores

Ancient Uses of Flaxseeds and Oil

Linseed oil has long been highly favored oil applied to wooden furniture. Customers were advised to purchase linseed oil at the hardware store and polish the teakwood with it about once or twice a year. It was a custom among farmers to coat their farm tools and implements with flaxseed oil to prevent rust.

After the oil is pressed from the flaxseeds, the remaining cake was sold to farmers as cattle feed. A mixture of honey and flaxseed oil was used as a remedy for removing unwanted spots on the face.

Linseed oil was incorporated as an emollient in making soap and as a drying agent in manufacturing printer's ink, artist's paints, and house paints. The linseed oil is also used in the commercial production of liniments for burns and joint pain. Many European farmers regularly feed their animals with flaxseeds to prevent as well as treat diseases.

Making of Flax Oil

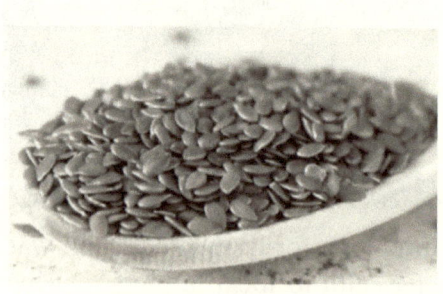

A special, cold-pressed and controlled expeller process that does not exceed temperatures of 96 F (36 C) in order to prevent damage produces truly high quality flax oil. Flax Oil spoils at 42 degree Celsius. Quality flax oil is easily recognized by its lack of odor and its delicate, almost flavorless taste. Some describe the taste of flaxseed oil as slightly nutty. To get the best quality oil the seeds should be organic and pressed only once. After expelling the oil should be packed in dark colored glass bottles with nitrogen flushed. Cold chain should be mentioned during transportation.

You should store the Flax oil in the freeze. You can safely use the oil for four months if you store it in refrigerator and for nine months if you keep in freezer section. But at room temperature oil is spoiled after one month. You should also protect the oil from light and air. The flax oil should never be heated.

The term expeller pressed involves a mechanical process of pressing the flaxseeds to make oil. Though product labels may say cold pressed, temperatures produced by this process that are not carefully controlled can reach as high as 200 F (93 C), even though no external heat is applied.

Nutrients Name	Nutrient Value	Percentage of RDA
Energy	534 Kcal	27%
Carbohydrates	28.8 g	22%
Protein	18.3 g	32.5%
Total Fat	42.16 g	170%
Dietary Fiber	27.3 g	68%
Vitamins		
Folates	87 µg	22%
Niacin	3.08 mg	19%
Pantothenic acid	0.985 mg	20%
Pyridoxine	0.473 mg	36%
Riboflavin	0.161 mg	12%
Thiamin	1.64 mg	137%
Vitamin C	0.6 mg	1%
Vitamin E	19.95 mg	133%
Vitamin K	4.3 µg	3.5%
Electrolytes		
Sodium	30 mg	2%
Potassium	813 mg	17%
Minerals		
Calcium	255 mg	22.5%
Copper	1.12 mg	124%
Iron	5.73 mg	72%
Magnesium	392 mg	98%
Manganese	2.48 mg	108%
Zinc	4.34 mg	39%
Phyto-nutrients		
Lutein-zeaxanthin	651 µg	--

Higher temperatures produce more oil though it is of a lesser quality because flax oil is highly polyunsaturated oil and can easily be damaged by heat, light, and exposure to air. In its damaged state, flax oil becomes tainted with toxic molecules called lipid peroxides that are harmful to the body. The telltale signs are a bitter taste and rancid odor.

Composition of flaxseed

Flaxseed is a highly nutritious food. Flaxseed contains the omega-3 fatty acid, alpha-linolenic acid (ALA), fiber and lignans. About 42% of flaxseed is oil and more than 70% of that oil is comprised of healthy polyunsaturated fatty acids. Flaxseed contains 55-57% of the essential omega-3 fatty acid, ALA.

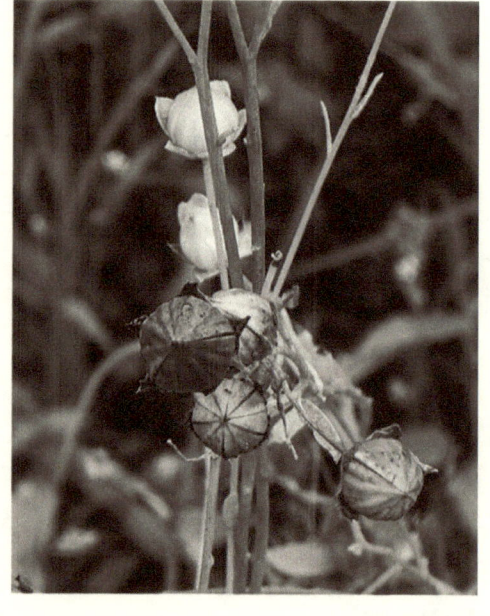

Flaxseed contains soluble as well as insoluble fiber. Soluble fiber can lower blood cholesterol levels and help lower blood sugar, while insoluble fiber moves the stool through the colon more quickly, helping bowel movements and improving evacuation.

Flaxseed is one of the richest plant sources of lignans, providing up to 800 times more lignans than most other foods. Lignans are phytoestrogens – compounds that have been shown to help protect against certain kinds of cancer, particularly cancers of the breast and colon.

How Linseed became Flaxseed??

Flaxseed oil is now of very popular and used by millions in Americans for its wonderful health benefits, thanks to two men who fought hard to bring this super oil to U.S.A. Less than 35 years ago, flaxseed was known as "linseed oil." The federal Food and Drug Administration declared that humans shouldn't use it because it was sold as a paint additive.

Mike Minarsich, founder of BioNatures in 1986, read a story about Dr. Johanna Budwig and her amazing work Oil-Protein Cookbook. He wanted to know more, so he searched for the raw, cold-pressed linseed (now flaxseed) oil – at health-food stores and companies. He contacted William Fischer, publisher of Dr. Budwig's book, and discovered that the German publisher had used "edible" linseed oil since he was a child.

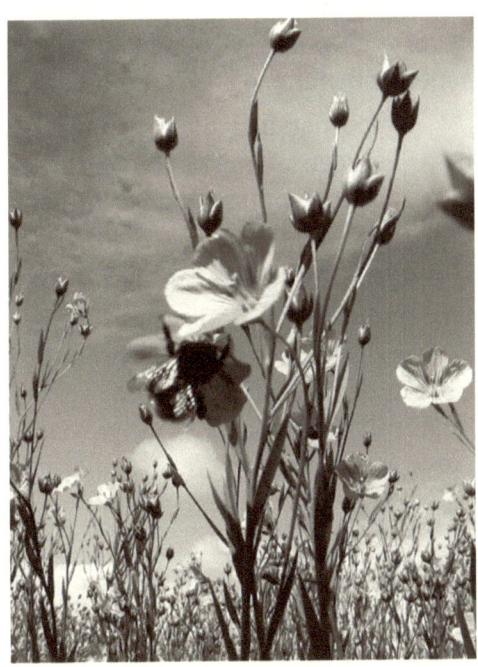

Then, Mike found a Canadian company that produced "linseed" oil according to the standards of Dr. Budwig.

And so he formed BioNatures Company. Bionatures was the first company in America to import and sell linseed oil for human use. Demand soared, in large part because of Fischer's landmark book. But soon the FDA stopped BioNatures' shipments at the Canadian border, claiming that linseed oil is a drying agent for paint and is not suitable for human consumption. BioNatures argued that THIS linseed oil was cold-pressed in a pharmaceutical facility for human consumption and was not the same linseed oil sold in hardware stores. The FDA still said no.

So they came up with two ideas: Find someone in the U.S. to make the product and change the name from linseed oil to flaxseed oil. After all, it was derived from plant that is called the flax plant. Eventually confusion for the government and consumers was eliminated and a partnership established between BioNatures and a young man in northern Washington State named Bruce Barlean and his father. Bruce and his family were fishermen who had vision. Already familiar with the health benefits of omega 3 oils from fish, they saw the potential for the superior benefits of flaxseed oil and byproducts.

Bruce pursued the new idea vigorously. With BioNatures' help, Barleans Organic Oils was born. It is now the country's largest manufacturer, thanks primarily to Bruce and Mike's will power and hard work.

Bruce Barlean made several trips to Germany to visit with Dr. Budwig, developed the proprietary Barlean's Bio-Electron Process TM, used today to produce the oil. It is the only process endorsed by Dr. Budwig. The rest is a history. Today if you type "flax oil" into google.com, you may get around 400,000 results. Now it is considered a staple item for most people's daily regimen (Minarsich).

Devotional Song of Goddess Linseed

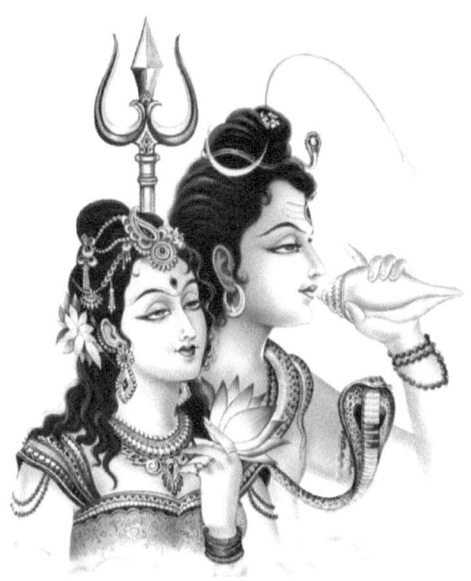

According to Hindu mythology Linseed Goddess is fifth incarnation of Holy Mother Durga. During ancient times Linseed Goddess was worshipped as Scand Mata on fifth day of Navratri festival and linseed was consumed as blessed food of Holy Mother. Linseed Goddess is also known as Parvati, Neelpushpi, Kshuma, Uma etc. Linseed is a panacea and balances vata, pitta and kapha all three doshas. The worshipper is blessed with health, vitality and divine power. He never gets sick throughout the year. All of his wishes are fulfilled. Linseed Goddess gives him eternal bliss and straight way opens the door of Moksha (Heaven).

This is a translation of devotion song of Godess Linseed.

In the Holly books following shloka are written in the praise of Linseed Goddess.

9

If Lord Shiva and Goddess Parvati are living together, the whole world would be happy and prosperous.

Golden ear pendant and sandal wood cream applied on her forehead is shining like moon.

Master of whole universe holding snake over his body dances with his fair Goddess.

Goddess Linseed is greatest among all other Goddesses, as she keeps everybody healthy and vibrant.

She is a fountain of youth and shines our nails, hair and whole body.

All old Monks say that anger goes away and happiness is achieved.

She supercharges your mind, gives you divine mental powers and flows channel of knowledge.

She is an anti-ageing elixir, cures ailments and has unlimited healing properties.

She is symbol of faith, devotion and love. She makes you blissful.

She helps in meditation, arouses your dormant serpent energy (Kundalini) and opens the doors of heaven.

This is the original shloka written ancient Hindu Holy books.

अलसी नीलपुष्पी पावर्तती स्यादुमा क्षुमा।

अलसी मधुरा तिक्ता स्निग्धापाके कदुर्गरु:॥

उष्णा दृष शुक वातन्धी कफ पित्त विनाशिनी।

Original Hindi bhajans (Devotional song) written for Goddess Linseed.

अलसी भजन

शंकर संग सुनंदा   भयो रे जग आनंदा
मस्तक चंदन कान के कुंडल   चमके जैसे चंदा
गौरा संग नाचे त्रिपुरारी लिपटे देह भुजंगा
सब देवियों में अलसी बड़ी है करदे सबको चंगा
तन में यौवन भर देती है चमके नख शिख अंगा
क्रोध न आए खुशियां लाए   कहते सारे महंता
सुमति जगाये सद्गुण आये बहती ज्ञान की गंगा
उम्र बढ़ाये रोग भगाये गुण है तेरे अनंता
श्रद्धा भक्ति प्रेम बढ़ाये तू ही परमानंदा
ध्यान लगाये कुंडलि जगाये छूटे जग का फंदा
धुन- नटवर नागर नंदा भजो रे मन..

अलसी मैया की आरती

आरती अलसी मैया   की
शशधिर रूप दुलारी की ॥
स्वास्थ्य की देवी कहलाती
भक्त की   पीड़ा हर लेती
मोक्ष के द्वार खोल देती
शत्रु हो त्रस्त
रोग हो ध्वस्त
देह हो स्वस्थ
दयामयी उमा सुनीला की
शशधिर रूप दुलारी की ॥

11

त्वचा में लाये कोमलता
कनक जैसी हो सुन्दरता
छलकता यौवन का सोता
बदन में महक
केश में चमक
वदन में दमक
मोहिनी नील कुमारी की
शशधिर रूप दुलारी की ॥
तुम्हीं हो करुणा का सागर
कृपा से भर दो तुम गागर
धन्य हो जाऊँ मैं पाकर
तू देती शक्ति
करूँ मैं भक्ति
दिला दे मुक्ति
उज्ज्वला मनोहारिणी की
शशधिर रूप दुलारी की ॥
ज्ञान और बुद्धि का वर दो
तेज और प्रतिभा से भर दो
ओम को दिव्य चक्षु दे दो
न जाऊं भटक
बिछाऊं पलक
दिखादे झलक
रुद्र प्रिय मतिवाहिनी की
शशधिर रूप दुलारी की ॥
क्रोध मद आलस को हर ले
हृदय को खुशियों से भर दे
आयु और ममता का वर दे
मची है धूम

मन रहा घूम
भक्त रहे झूम
स्कंद मां पालनहारी की
शशधिर रूप दुलारी की ॥
धुन- आरती कुंज बिहारी की..

Flaxseed – Storehouse of Essential Fats

Fatty acid is a carboxylic acid with a long unbranched aliphatic carbon chain, which is either saturated or unsaturated. Most natural occurring fatty acids have a chain of 4 to 28 carbons. There is always even number of carbons. First Carbon from carboxyl end is called α, second β, third γ, fourth δ .…. And last carbon is called ω or omega and the last end is called omega end.

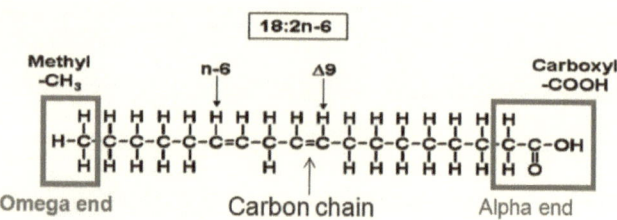

Chain Length of Fatty Acids

Very Long chain FA 23 – 28 Carbons - A very long chain fatty acid (VLCFA) is a fatty acid with aliphatic tails longer than 22 carbons. Unlike most fatty acids, VLCFAs are too long to be metabolized in the mitochondria, and must be metabolized in peroxisomes.

Long chain FA 13 – 22 Carbons - are most important fatty acids for us like ALA, LA, EPA, DHA etc.

Medium chain FA 6 - 12 Carbons - MCTs are caproic acid (C6), caprylic acid (C8), capric acid (C10) and lauric acid (C12). Coconut oil is composed of approximately 66% medium-chain fatty acids.

Short chain FA 4 - 6 Carbons - like Formic acid, Propionic acid, Isobutyric acid, Butyric acid, Isovaleric acid & valeric acid. These are produced in the large bowel as a result of bacterial fermentation of soluble fiber.

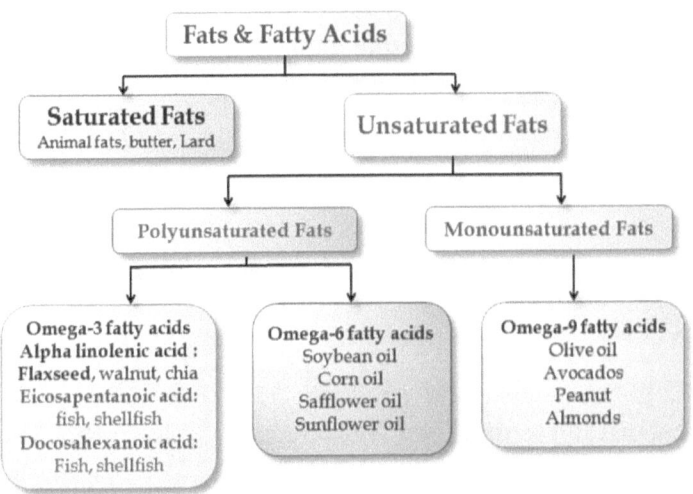

```
Fats & Fatty Acids
    |
    |------------------------|
    |                        |
Saturated Fats         Unsaturated Fats
Animal fats, butter, Lard        |
                    |--------------------|
                    |                    |
          Polyunsaturated Fats    Monounsaturated Fats
                    |                    |
          |-------------|               |
```

Omega-3 fatty acids Alpha linolenic acid : Flaxseed, walnut, chia Eicosapentanoic acid: fish, shellfish Docosahexanoic acid: Fish, shellfish	Omega-6 fatty acids Soybean oil Corn oil Safflower oil Sunflower oil	Omega-9 fatty acids Olive oil Avocados Peanut Almonds

Alpha-Linolenic Acid ALA

- Short Formula   18:3 n-3
- That means it has a chain of 18 carbons, 3 sis double bonds and first double bond is located after 3rd carbon from omega end.
- Melting point (-)11 degree Celsius

Alpha-Linolenic Acid (ALA)

Docosahexanoic acid DHA

- Short Formula   22:6 n-3
- That means it has a chain of 22 carbons, 6 sis double bonds and first double bond is located after 3rdcarbon as usual.
- Melting point (-)50 degree Celsius

Eicosapentaanoic acid EPA

- Short Formula   20:5 n-3

- That means it has a chain of 20 carbons, 5 sis double bonds and first double bond is located after 3rd carbon as usual.
- Melting point (-)56 degree Celsius

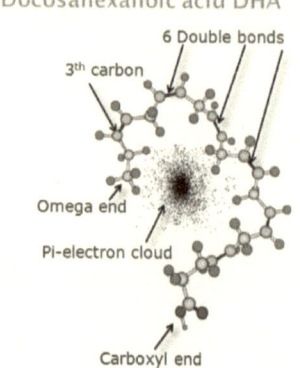

Docosahexanoic acid DHA

6 Double bonds

3th carbon

Omega end

Pi-electron cloud

Carboxyl end

Dietary source of EPA and DHA

Cold water fish and shellfish - salmon, sardines, mackerel, herring, and tuna.

Functions of omega-3

- Anti-clotting (thrombolytic) effect – acts as Natural Aspirin
- Lowering the risk of heart disease – heart attack (Coronary Artery Disease) and atherosclerosis
- Lowering triglycerides in the blood
- Lowering high blood pressure
- Reduction in heart irregularities – Arrhythmia.
- Helping to alleviate mood disorders, such as depression. Reducing aggression
- Helping patients with attention deficit/hyperactivity disorder (ADHD), dyslexia and dyspraxia
- Helping to improve memory and learning skills, and prevent Alzheimer's disease
- Improves immunity and Alleviates allergic disorders
- Improving inflammatory skin disorders such as psoriasis and eczema
- Alleviating osteoarthritis, gout and rheumatoid arthritis (RA)
- Alleviating Pre Menstrual Syndrome PMS

- Alleviating Menopausal Symptoms – Hot flushes, dry vagina, mood swing
- Improvement of vision

Linoleic Acid LA

- Short Formula - 18:2 n-6
- That means it has a chain of 18 carbons, 2 sis double bonds and first double bond is located after 6th carbon from omega end
- Melting point (-)5 degree Celsius

Arachidonic Acid AA

- Short Formula 20:4 n-6
- That means it has a chain of 20 carbons, 4 sis double bonds and first double bond is located after 6th carbon from omega end.
- Food sources - butter, animal fats, especially pork, organ meats, eggs and seaweed.

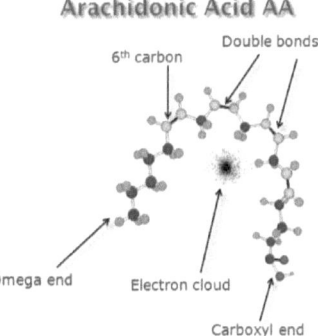

Cis and Trans configuration

The two carbon atoms in the chain that are bound next to either side of the double bond can occur in a cis or Trans configuration.

Cis configuration

- Cis configuration means that adjacent hydrogen atoms are on the same side of the double bond.

- The cis configuration causes the chain to bend by 350 and cis fatty acids are thermodynamically less stable than the Trans forms.
- The cis fatty acids have lower melting points than the Trans fatty acids or their saturated counterparts.
- Cis fats have live, energy rich electrons
- Sis and natural Essential fats are rich in live, energy rich electrons.
- Electrons are key to health and longevity. This is biggest "Anti-entropy Factor".
- Electrons are extremely important to the body's overall energy exchange potential "the flow of life force."

Trans fats — Trans double bond — No electrons

Vital sis fats — Sis double bond — Live energy rich electrons

Tran's configuration

- A Tran's configuration, by contrast, means that the next two hydrogen atoms are bound to opposite sides of the double bond.
- As a result, they do not cause the chain to bend, and their shape is similar to straight saturated fatty acids.
- Most fatty acids in the Trans configuration (Tran's fats) are not found in nature and are the result of human processing (e.g., hydrogenation).

Trans Fats – The deadly fats

- Increase cancer risk factors.
- Elevate cardiovascular risk factors.
- Interfere with insulin function.
- Decrease testosterone.
- Change the fluidity of cell membranes.
- Interfere with the healing fats.
- Trans fats are "anti-human", electron-poor, directed into the past, life functions are paralyzed, lacks energy and

strength because the electrons that are in harmony with the sun as "life-element" are missing.
- Tran's fat is the biggest enemy of mankind.

Prostaglandins - Overview

- Localized tissue hormones.
- They do not travel in the blood like hormones.
- Prostaglandins are potent but have a short life and are either locally active (Paracrine) or act on the same cell (Autocrine) within which they are synthesized.
- The prostaglandins perform different functions in the body.

Good and Bad Prostaglandins

Good Prostaglandins	Bad Prostaglandins
Decreased platelet aggregation (prevents blood clotting)	Increased platelet aggregation (helps in blood clotting)
Vasodilatation (widening of blood vessels)	Vasoconstriction (narrowing of vessels)
Anti-inflammatory effect	Pro-inflammatory effect
Immune system enhancement	Immune system suppression
Increased oxygen flow	Decreased oxygen flow
Decreased cell proliferation	Increased cell proliferation
Decreased pain	Increased pain
Widening of respiratory passages	Narrowing of respiratory passages
Increased endurance	Lowered endurance

Good – Anti-inflammatory
Series 3 prostaglandins

Series 1 prostaglandins

Bad – Pro-inflammatory
Series 2 prostaglandins

Prostaglandins - Functions

- Cause constriction or dilatation of blood vessels.
- Cause aggregation or disaggregation of platelets.
- Sensitize spinal neurons to pain.
- Constrict smooth muscle.
- Regulate inflammatory mediation.
- Regulate movement of calcium and other minerals & nutrients in the cell.
- Control hormone regulation.
- Control cell growth.
- Regulates cellular communication.

Series 3 prostaglandins

- The Series 3 prostaglandins are formed at a slower rate and work to attenuate excessive Series 2 production. Their response is "less vigorous".
- The omega-3 pathway might therefore be likened to the "slow lane".
- Adequate production of the Series 3 prostaglandins seems to protect against heart attack and stroke as well as certain inflammatory diseases like arthritis, lupus and asthma.

Series 1 prostaglandins

- Series 1 prostaglandins are Anti-inflammatory, Thrombolytic - Decreased platelet aggregation (blood clotting), pain reliever and control cellular activities.
- The strong anti-inflammatory properties help the body recover from injury by reducing pain, swelling and redness.

Series 2 prostaglandins

- Series 2 PG seem to be involved in swelling inflammation, clotting and dilation.
- Series 2 prostaglandins are "fast lane" i.e. involved in intense actions and play a role in swelling and

inflammation at sites of injury. This is not at all a "bad" effect, but an important protective mechanism - the body's way of immobilizing the affected site to prevent further injury and facilitate healing.

- Series 2 prostaglandins also seem to play a role in inducing birth, in regulating temperature, in lowering blood pressure, and in the regulation of platelet aggregation and clotting.

Omega-6 / Omega-3 Metabolic Pathways

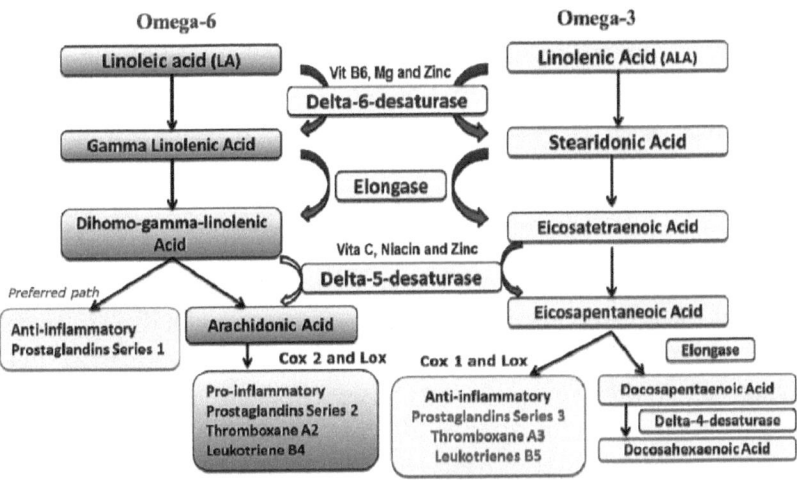

Prepared by Dr. O.P.Verma

Omega-6 / Omega-3 Metabolic Pathways

Although most omega-3 and omega-6 fatty acids are generally referred to as "essential" fatty acids, only linoleic acid (LA) of the omega-6 family and alpha-linolenic acid (ALA) of the omega-3 family are truly "essential". Once we have either LA or ALA, our body has enzymes that can convert these fatty acids into all the other different types of omega-6 and omega-3 fatty acids.

It turns out that both the omega-3 and omega-6 pathway utilize the same enzymes, and both omega-6 and omega-3 fatty acids have to compete for these enzymes in order to produce their final product. Studies have reported that the enzymes used in these pathways were found to prefer the omega-3 pathway. It turns out then that in diets high in omega-3 fatty acids, most of the enzymes will be "busy" converting the omega-3 acids.

The omega-6 fatty acids, Dihommogamma-Linoleic Acid (DGLA)) in particular, can be converted to either the anti-inflammatory PG1 or into arachidonic acid (AA), a precursor of PG2. Conversion of DGLA into PG1 does not require any enzymes, but conversion of DGLA into AA requires the enzyme delta-5 desaturase. In diets high in omega-3, most of the delta-5 desaturase will be used in the omega-3 pathway; few delta-5 desaturase will be available to convert DGLA into arachidonic acid, and subsequently, PG2. DGLA ends up being converted into the anti-inflammatory PG1 and inflammation is therefore decreased.

In a diet low in omega-3 fatty acids, large quantities of delta-5 desaturase enzymes are available to convert DGLA into AA. The available AA is then converted into the inflammatory PG2. Thus, the more omega-3 fatty acids present in our body, the fewer enzymes are available for converting omega-6 fatty acids into the inflammatory prostaglandins. A balance of omega-6 and omega-3 fatty acids is therefore essential for proper health. However, the typical Western diet has evolved to be high in omega-6 and low in omega-3 fatty acids. While omega-6 fatty acids are not necessarily bad, a skewed ratio in favor of too much omega-6 can be detrimental to one's health.

Balanced N-6/N-3 ratio – road to health, Ultra wellness & longevity

Balanced N-6/N-3 ratio

road to health, Ultra wellness & longevity

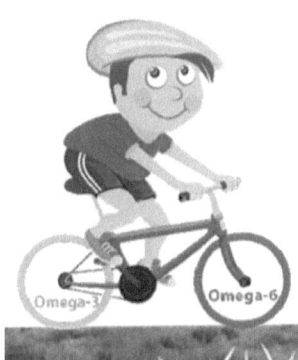

Road to health & longevity...

Both groups of prostaglandins perform vitally important functions and supplement each other through complex and multi-faceted interactions. For centuries ratio of Omega-6 and Omega-3 was perfect e.g. 2:1 or even 4:1 (very ideal ratio).

N-6/N-3 ratio out of balance - road to aging, disease & death

But after the global switch to industrial agriculture and processed foods it is 20:1 or more (!!!).

This throws the body into the state of chronic inflammation, giving rise to a whole array of clot and inflammation-related chronic diseases, including thrombosis, arthritis, diabetes, atherosclerosis and coronary heart disease (CHD, cancer and asthma.

There is only one crucial condition that must be fulfilled if the entire system is to work well and promote health, rather than disease. This condition is B A L A N C E.

N-6/N-3 ratio out of balance - road to aging, disease & death

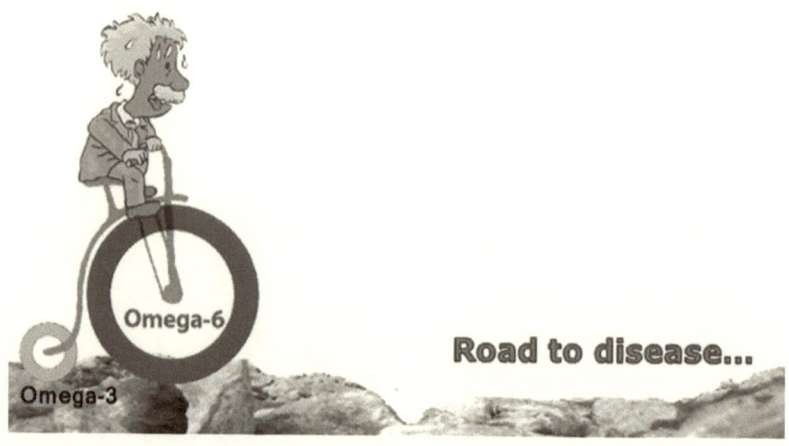

For the prostaglandin pathways to run smoothly, the intake of omega-3 and omega-6 fatty acids must be well-balanced, within the 1:2 to 4:1 range.

Risk of eating fish

- Fish is contaminated with deadly poisons like mercury, dioxins, polychlorinated biphenyls (PCBs), and pesticide residues.
- Very high levels of mercury can damage nerves in adults and disrupt development of the brain.

Benefits of eating flaxseed

- Flaxseed has much more Omega-3 than fish. Flaxseed had Alpha-linolenic acid, which is essential fatty acid and has ability to make all other omega-3's our body needs.
- There is no risk of mercury contamination.
- Flaxseed also provides us lot of fabulous fiber, legend lignans, magic minerals like selenium, zinc, Mg, potassium and vitamins. You get all this without killing a creature.

Metabolism of ALA

Alpha-linolenic acid (ALA) constitutes about 57% of the total fatty acids in flax, making flax one of the richest sources of ALA in the diet. Metabolism of ALA and its role in human health is described below.

ALA - True Essential Omega-3 Fatty Acid

ALA is the head of the omega-3 fatty acid family. It must be obtained from our diets because our bodies cannot make it. So, ALA is an essential nutrient just like vitamin C and calcium.

ALA Is Needed for Good Health

ALA has important functions in our body and helps prevent and manage chronic diseases like heart disease, stroke, type 2 diabetes, osteoarthritis and certain types of cancer. ALA calms down chronic inflammation, which is a key feature of many life style diseases, and it helps promote the proper functioning of blood vessels, which reduces the risk of heart attacks and stroke.

ALA constitutes 75-80% of total omega-3 fatty acids in breast milk that shows its importance for infant growth and development. ALA is also required for maintaining the nervous system. A deficiency of ALA in humans causes poor growth, depression, pain in the legs, difficulty walking and blurred vision. These deficiency symptoms can be subsided by adding ALA to the diet.

Metabolic Fates of ALA

Dietary ALA has several metabolic fates. This is how ALA is used by our body.

- Increases the omega-3 fat content of cell membranes. ALA is incorporated into the triglycerides and phospholipids of cell membranes, where it affects how nutrients are transferred into and out of the cell and how cells communicate with one another. Increasing the omega-3 content of cell membranes makes them more flexible and decreases inflammation.

- Is converted to long-chain omega-3 fatty acids. ALA is converted to the long-chain omega-3 fatty acids, particularly EPA and docosapentaenoic acid (DPA).
- Produces energy. ALA undergoes ß-oxidation to produce energy for the work of muscles, the digestion of food, breathing, and the like. About 24-33% of an ingested dose of ALA undergoes ß-oxidation in men; in women.
- Is used to make ketone bodies. ALA appears to be preferred over linoleic acid (an omega-6 fatty acid) as a substrate for ketogenesis – the process of making ketone bodies. Ketone bodies serve as an alternate energy source for the brain during starvation or fasting. This function of ALA may be important in maintaining healthy cognition in elderly adults.
- Is stored for future energy needs. ALA is stored in adipose tissue, where it serves as a reserve supply of energy. Women store more ALA in their adipose tissue than men because of their greater fat mass.

ALA Metabolism

The metabolic pathways of the omega-3 and omega-6 fatty acids are shown in the figure below. The discussion that follows focuses on the metabolism of the omega-3 family of fatty acids.

Desaturation and elongation. ALA is converted to long-chain fatty acids by a series of alternating desaturations and elongations. The desaturations add a double bond by removing hydrogen, while the elongations add two carbon atoms.

The first step in ALA metabolism is desaturation, catalyzed by delta-6-desaturase. This step is considered rate-limiting, as it is most affected by nutritional, hormonal and metabolic factors.

The desaturation and elongation steps occur in the endoplasmic reticulum of the cell. The desaturation steps tend to be slow, while the elongation steps are rapid. For this reason, the tissue concentration of stearidonic acid tends to be low, because it is formed slowly by desaturation and then quickly elongated to other metabolites.

26

Competition between fatty acid families. Mammals cannot interconvert the omega-3 and omega-6 fatty acids. That is, omega-3 fatty acids cannot be changed into omega-6 fatty acids, or vice versa. Furthermore, there is competition between the two families. An excess of one family of fatty acids can interfere with the metabolism of the other, changing their concentrations in tissues and their biological effects .

Efficiency of Conversion of ALA. Estimates of the conversion of ALA to EPA range from 0.2% to 8%, with young women showing a conversion rate as high as 21%. Conversion of ALA to DPA is estimated at 0.13% to 6%, with women showing a conversion rate on the higher end (6%).

Here again, young women appear to convert more ALA to DHA than men do – as much as 9% of ingested ALA may be converted to DHA in young women. A diet rich in linoleic acid decreases ALA conversion by as much as 40%. Saturated fat, oleic acid, Tran's fatty acids, and dietary cholesterol interfere with ALA desaturation and elongation. High intakes of EPA and DHA – and even of ALA itself – can decrease the conversion rate.

Lignans - 7 Star Nutrient of the Millennium

Lignans represent one of the four major classes of chemical compounds collectively known as phytoestrogens.

Phytoestrogens are plant chemicals that can have estrogen-like actions in humans. The main phytoestrogens are lignans, isoflavonoids, flavonoids and stilbenes. Their health benefits extend beyond

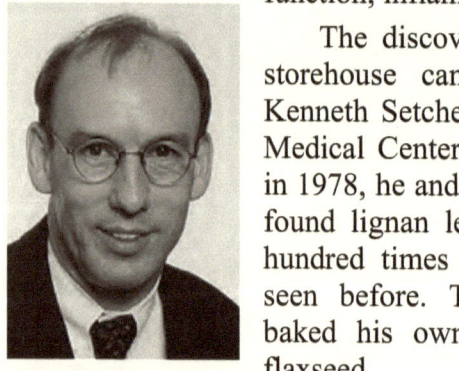

Lignans

hormone-dependent breast cancer, osteoporosis, and prostate cancer to include brain function, cardiovascular disease, immune function, inflammation and reproduction.

The discovery of flaxseed as a lignan storehouse came by sheer chance says Kenneth Setchell, PhD, Children's Hospital Medical Center, and Cincinnati. In a study in 1978, he and his colleagues unexpectedly found lignan levels in one patient several hundred times higher than had ever been seen before. The patient, it turned out, baked his own bread and always added flaxseed.

Flax Lignans

Flax is the richest source of plant lignans, being very rich in the lignan secoisolariciresinol diglucoside (SDG). Flax contains other lignans as well – namely, matairesinol, pinoresinol, lariciresinol, isolariciresinol and secoisolariciresinol (often abbreviated SECO).

The lignans SDG, SECO, pinoresinol, lariciresinol and matairesinol in flax are converted by bacteria in the colon to the mammalian lignans, enterodiol and enterolactone. Isolariciresinol is not converted to mammalian lignans. Enterodiol and enterolactone are called mammalian lignans or enterolignans because they are produced in the gut of humans; they are not found in plants. The biologic activity of flax lignans depends on the presence of certain bacteria in the gut. Lignans in flaxseeds are 47 to 800 times more than any other lignan source. Gram for gram, flax has 47 times the total lignan content of sesame seeds and more than 600 times the total lignan content of garlic. Whole flax seed contains 1-26 mg SDG/g, which works out to about 11-286 mg SDG/tbsp of whole seed.

Foodstuff	Secoisolariciresinol	
Flaxseed	**165759**	µg / 100 g
Sesame seeds	240	µg / 100 g
Rye bran	462	µg / 100 g
Wheat bran	868	µg / 100 g
Oat bran	90	µg / 100 g
Barley bran	42	µg / 100 g

Nectar of Rejuvenation

Flax lignans and the mammalian lignans (enterodiol and enterolactone) are biologically active. Lignans have antibacterial, antifungal, antiviral, anti-lupus, anti-allergic, anti-HIV and anticancer properties. They influence gene expression and may protect against estrogen-related diseases such as breast cancer and osteoporosis. Diets high in lignans may help maintain good cognitive function in post-menopausal women; reduce breast cancer risk in women and reduce the risk of acute fatal coronary events and prostate cancer in men.

The main flax lignan SDG is a powerful antioxidant. It scavenges for certain free radicals like the hydroxyl ion (•OH). Our bodies produce free radicals continually as we metabolize fats, proteins, alcohol and some carbohydrates for energy. Free radicals can damage tissues and have been implicated in the pathology of many diseases like atherosclerosis, cancer and Alzheimer disease. The mammalian lignans, enterodiol and enterolactone, also act as antioxidants. Indeed, the antioxidant action of SECO and enterodiol is five times greater than that of vitamin E.

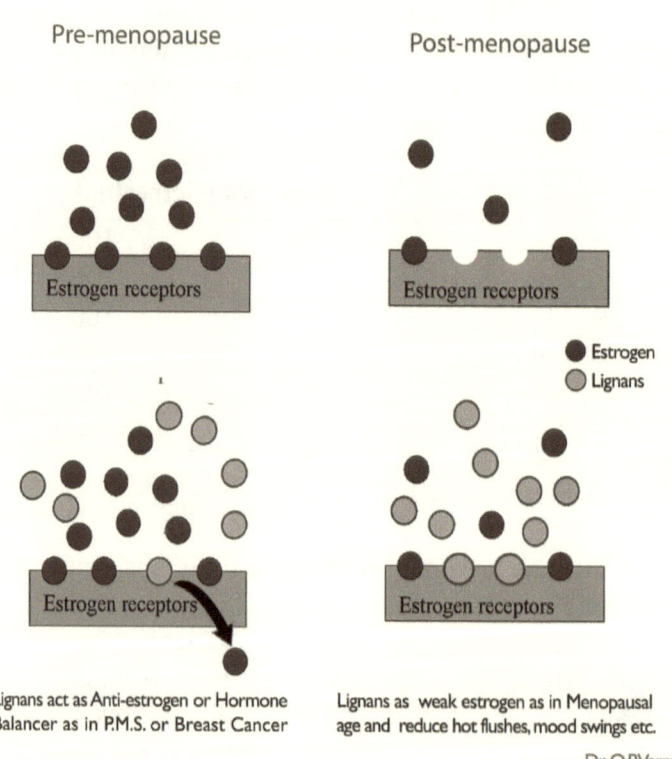

Lignans - Mode of Action

Pre-menopause   Post-menopause

● Estrogen
○ Lignans

Lignans act as Anti-estrogen or Hormone Balancer as in P.M.S. or Breast Cancer

Lignans as weak estrogen as in Menopausal age and reduce hot flushes, mood swings etc.

Dr. O.P.Verma

Lignan favorably influences immune reactions. ALA and lignans block the release of pro-inflammatory cytokines and decrease blood CRP levels. Lignans have been shown to decrease the production of TNFα and IL-6. Lignans are Platelet activating factor receptor antagonists and thus block the pro-inflammatory actions of PAF. Through these effects, flax consumption may help prevent and treat disorders characterized in part by an over-stimulated immune system. Such disorders include obesity, metabolic syndrome, rheumatoid arthritis, multiple sclerosis and systemic lupus erythematosus (SLE). The researchers concluded that a flax lignan taken daily resulted in a modest improvement in sugar control in the adults with type 2 diabetes.

Relative antioxidant activity	
Vitamin E	1
SDG (Flax lignan)	1.27
SECO (aglycone)	4.86
Enterodiol (mammalian lignan)	5.02
Enterolactone (mammalian lignan)	4.35

Lignans - Elixir of Womanhood

It is hypothesized that the interplay between natural estrogen and lignans, is a prerequisite for optimal health in women. Therefore, they have a plethora of positive roles to play in women's health issues. Estrogen levels are typically high in women during the childbearing years and then fall away through the post-menopausal years. While lignans have estrogen-like action, they are considerably weaker than our endogenous estrogen, and act as hormone balancers. An important feature of these plant hormones is that they do not stimulate reproductive tissue. In conditions which are linked with excess estrogen (such as PMS, osteoporosis, unhealthy breast tissue and breast cancer) lignans compete with a woman's own estrogen, having an estrogen lowering effect.

In conditions associated with declining estrogen levels such as menopause, lignans have the opposite effect. This balancing action is due to their ability to competitively lock onto our body's Estrogen receptor sites. Consequently, lignans are used to reduce symptoms of menopause, such as hot flushes, night sweats, mood swings and breast tenderness. Lignans have beneficial effects on the menstrual cycle. They reduce the risk of uterine fibroids in middle-aged women.

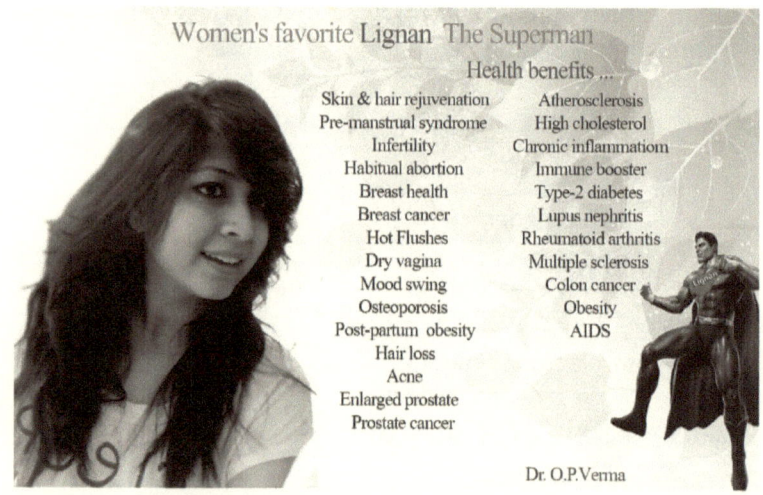

Women's favorite Lignan The Superman

Health benefits ....

Skin & hair rejuvenation
Pre-manstrual syndrome
Infertility
Habitual abortion
Breast health
Breast cancer
Hot Flushes
Dry vagina
Mood swing
Osteoporosis
Post-partum obesity
Hair loss
Acne
Enlarged prostate
Prostate cancer

Atherosclerosis
High cholesterol
Chronic inflammatiom
Immune booster
Type-2 diabetes
Lupus nephritis
Rheumatoid arthritis
Multiple sclerosis
Colon cancer
Obesity
AIDS

Dr. O.P.Verma

Lignan has been found to substantially increase milk production in women who are not producing enough milk to nurse their infants. Lignans may shape up small and loose breasts in young women. These days women put weight after her first delivery. Lignans prevent this post-delivery obesity.

Heart friendly

Today people are turning to more natural ingredients to maintain overall heart health and reduce risk factors to the heart. Cardiovascular disease is the result of atherosclerosis, in which deposits of cholesterol and other substances accumulate and form plaque on artery walls. Plaque build-up can gradually narrow the lumen of the artery, restricting blood flow. Sometimes plaque breaks away from the artery wall, which can cause a blood clot. A heart attack or stroke can occur when blood flow is completely blocked. High cholesterol is a risk factor for cardiovascular disease. Free radicals are also implicated in the development of atherosclerosis or hardening of the artery walls. Studies suggest that the dietary fiber and certain fatty acids in flax can help reduce risks of cardiovascular disease. Research also suggests that flax lignans play a major role in cardiovascular health. The effectiveness of SDG in heart health could be due to their powerful antioxidant activity. Lignans block the oxidation of LDL particles and decreasing their deposition in arterial walls. The oxidation of LDL is believed to be a key pathological event in the development of atherosclerosis. Flaxseed taken daily can reduce total and bad (LDL) cholesterol levels, whole flaxseed contains several heart health components (fatty acids, fiber and lignans). These studies could not tell us how much effect is due to the lignans.

Cancer killer

Mammalian lignans appear to exert anticancer effects through both hormone and non-hormone-related actions. The mammalian lignans enterodiol and enterolactone inhibit two key enzymes involved in estrogen synthesis; both enzymes are associated with increased breast cancer risk. Lignans may also have non-hormone-related actions, such as antioxidant activity, inhibiting angiogenesis (the growth of blood vessels that supply oxygen and nutrients to tumors for growth), cell proliferation and promote cancer cell apoptosis (destruction) and/or altering the expression of growth factors that stimulate tumor 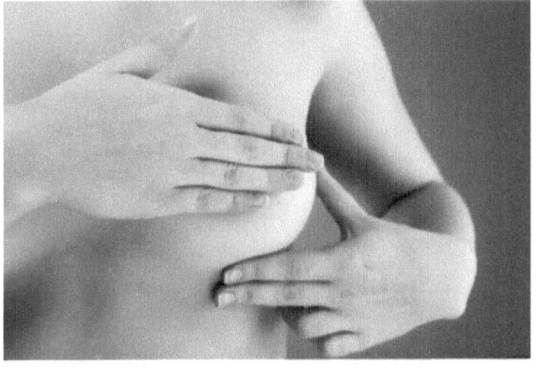 development. Cancer cells utilize the tyrosine kinase enzymes to fuel their rapid growth. Enterolactone helps to inhibit the tyrosine kinase enzyme.

Acne

Millions of people suffer from acne, a condition affecting the pilosebaceous units of skin. During puberty, the production of adrenal androgens is increased in both boys and girls. The elevation of androgens can cause an increase in sebum production, particularly in the face (sebum is a waxy substance that helps the skin retains moisture). Excess sebum can lead to acne.

Hormone related conditions

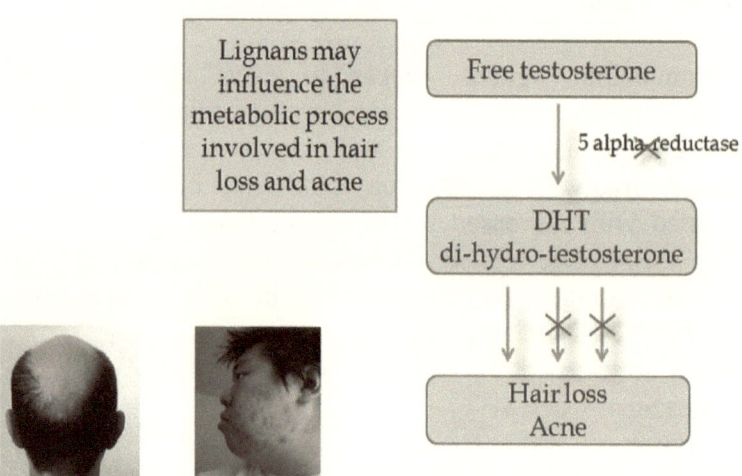

Lignans have been shown to inhibit 5 alpha-reductase, an enzyme involved in the conversion of testosterone to DHT. Inhibition of this enzyme shows promise in the treatment of a number of androgen-dependent disorders, including acne. Therefore flax lignans are definitely the perfect treatment of acne.

Baldness

Androgenetic alopecia the most common form of hair loss, is a hormonal as well as a genetic issue. Dihydrotestosterone (DHT), a potent form of the male hormone testosterone, can get inside hair follicles and make them shrink so that they produce thinner hair and eventually none at all. Secoisolariciresinol diglucoside (SDG), the main flax lignan, can help prevent this by inhibiting production of the enzyme that converts testosterone into DHT, called 5-alpha reductase. Thus lignans are very miraculous for hair growth.

Protector of manhood

Flax lignans have many potential benefits for men, specifically in prostate health. A great deal of attention is being focused on benign prostatic hyperplasia (BPH). This condition can be a problem because the urethra, the tube carrying urine from the bladder to outside the body, runs through the prostate. A growing prostate can pinch off the urethra and cause uncomfortable symptoms, like a frequent and overwhelming urge to urinate and painful urination. The exact cause of BPH is unknown but male hormones seem to play a role. Hormones also play a role in another prostate condition - prostate cancer, the second leading cause of cancer death among men.

In the body, testosterone is converted to a more potent form called dihydrotestosterone or DHT. Normal, healthy prostate cells require DHT for growth. However, it is thought that too much of the hormone can cause abnormal growth— leading to an 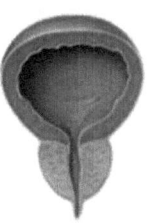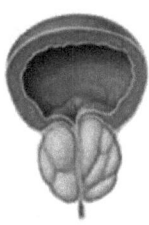 enlarged prostate (BPH) or causing prostate cancer cells to divide. Therefore, prostate health depends on balanced levels of these hormones. Lignans are shown to block the action of the enzyme (5 alpha- reductase) that converts testosterone into the more potent form (DHT).

Additionally, lignans have also been shown to inhibit other enzymes, which are essential for the synthesis of testosterone and estrogen. Lignans may also potentially reduce the amount of free testosterone available for the body to use. In the average male, only a small amount of testosterone roams free in the blood. Most testosterone is bound to protein called sex hormone binding globulin (SHBG). An increase in SHBG would theoretically leave less testosterone available to stimulate prostate cell growth. Lignans have been shown to increase SHBG production. Lignans also lower prostate specific antigen (PSA) levels (a marker for prostate cancer).

New hope to AIDS patients

Dear Doctors,

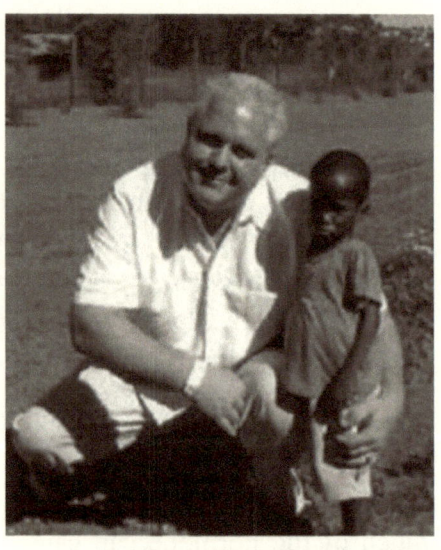

I am thrilled to tell you about miracle treatment (Flax Lignans) for AIDS patients. The Flax Lignans supercharge the depleted immune system and gives an AIDS sufferer a new life, new hope and a future. All it takes is for an AIDS patient to have the lignans in their system for 6-12 weeks to see their viral loads drop and their CD-4 counts skyrocket. We even have kids who have been on it for several years who are declared HIV negative now. Flax Lignan cost pennies per day for a child with AIDS.

Dr. Danial Daves, Director,
AIDS Research
Assistance Institute

Why should you take a lignan dietary supplement?

Most of us don't eat enough unrefined grains, fruits, vegetables, nuts and legumes necessary to provide the plant lignans we need to benefit our health. The average intake of lignans in India is only about 1 milligram per day. Yet, researchers say that we need a minimum of 50 to 100 milligrams of lignans per day in order to raise our enterolactone levels. To get enough lignan you should consume 1 scoop of milled flax, 54.8 Kg broccoli, 59 Kg garlic, 83 Kg soybeans, 118 Kg carrots or 2248 Kg oat meal.

Studies done so far indicate that dietary Phytoestrogens exert positive, balancing and protective effects in humans. In the past 18 months, consumer awareness of plant lignans has grown tremendously with media coverage of studies proposing its health benefits. In past few years lot of research has been done but still tons of information is in the pipeline. Today we admire flaxseeds as a great source of omega-3 fats but tomorrow it will be remembered as the greatest source of nutritional superman - The L i g n a n.

Funda of Fabulous fiber

The word fiber can also be spelled fibre (British). It comes from the Latin word fibra, meaning fiber, thread, string or filament. The most authentic definition of fiber available in medical literature is as follows.

"Dietary fiber is the edible parts of plants or analogous carbohydrates that are resistant to digestion and absorption in the human small intestine with complete or partial fermentation in the large intestine. Dietary fiber includes polysaccharides, oligosaccharides, lignin, and associated plant substances. Dietary fibers promote beneficial physiological effects including laxation, and/or blood cholesterol attenuation, and/or blood glucose attenuation."

Constituents of Dietary Fiber

Non-Starch Polysaccharides and Resistant Oligosaccharides
- Cellulose
- Hemicellulose
  - Arabinoxylans
  - Arabinogalactans
- Polyfructoses
  - Inulin
  - Oligofructans
- Galactooligosaccharides
- Gums
- Mucilages
- Pectins

Analogous Carbohydrates

- Indigestible Dextrins
  - o Resistant Maltodextrins (from corn and other sources)
  - o Resistant Potato Dextrins
- Synthesized Carbohydrate Compounds
  - o Polydextrose
  - o Methyl cellulose
  - o Hydroxypropylmethyl Cellulose
- Indigestible ("resistant") Starches

Lignin

Substances Associated with the Non-Starch Polysaccharide and Lignin Complex in Plants

- Waxes
- Phytate
- Cutin
- Saponins
- Suberin
- Tannins

Soluble fiber

Soluble fiber dissolves in water. It is readily fermented in the colon into gases and physiologically active byproducts and can be prebiotic and viscous. Soluble fibers tend to slow the movement of food through the system.

Soluble fiber has many benefits, including moderating blood glucose levels and lowering cholesterol. The scientific names for soluble fibers include pectins, gums, mucilages, and some hemicelluloses. Good sources of soluble fiber include oats and oatmeal, legumes (peas, beans, lentils), barley, fruits and vegetables (especially oranges, apples and carrots).

Benefits of Soluble Fiber are as follows:

- Reduce **heart disease** risk
- Regulate blood sugars through the fiber and Omega-3 essential fatty acids
- Promote growth of friendly flora
- **Soothe** irritable bowel
- **Lower total cholesterol**, the BAD cholesterol - LDL and has been shown to help reduce risk of **heart disease**
- Help people with **Diabetes** control their blood sugars better

Insoluble fiber

Insoluble fiber does not absorb or dissolve in water. It passes through our digestive system in close to its original form. Insoluble fiber offers many benefits to intestinal health, including a reduction in the risk and occurrence of hemorrhoids and constipation. The scientific names for insoluble fibers include cellulose, lignins, and also some other hemicelluloses. Most of insoluble fibers come from the bran layers of cereal grains.

Insoluble fiber is metabolically inert and provides bulking, or it can be prebiotic and metabolically ferment in the large intestine. Bulking fibers absorb water as they move through the digestive system, easing evacuation. Insoluble fibers tend to accelerate the movement of food through the system.

- Prevent and Relieve Constipation as well as diarrhea
- **Cleanse, Soothe and Heal** the colon
- Promotes **regular** bowel movements
- Keeps **toxins, cholesterol and waste** moving out of the colon
- Help to **balance the acidity** of the intestines
- Help promote optimal pH in colon which can prevent colon cancer

- The insoluble fiber exercises the bowel muscles as it helps broom out debris from the colon and provides bulk for the formation of feces.

Mucilage

Flax Mucilage is a type of Soluble Fiber that is **important for protecting and healing the colon.** It is a thick, gelatinous substance that swells as it absorbs water. Benefits of Mucilage on Health are as follows:

- An **emollient to help soothe, soften, heal tissue** and promotes regular bowel movements, which **prevents toxicity** and help **decrease bad LDL cholesterol**
- A **demulcent**, which **soothes, protects and heals** the internal tissues of the body including the intestines from irritation and inflammation
- Helps promote good flora in the gut which protects us from the harmful bacteria
- Helps to decrease or eliminate food cravings that come from **low blood sugar** and the body's need for good fats and fiber - this helps maintain good blood sugars and maintain healthy weight.
- **Reduces irritation of the gut**, which is especially beneficial for people who have IBS (irritable bowel), diverticulosis, and other intestinal problems.

The recommended fiber intake is 20 - 35 grams per day for adults, or 10 - 13 grams for every 1,000 calories in the diet. This recommended amount should come from a combination of soluble and insoluble fiber, since each type provides different benefits.

Constipation

For millions of people, constipation is a disorder they battle daily. Constipation has **immeasurable health risks** as fecal matter sitting in the colon can prevent the body from being able to get rid of toxins and waste material our body does not want.

Flaxseed helps relieve constipation with its Omega 3 oils as well as the healing and soothing mucilage fiber. It is important to drink water after eating flaxseed because it will swell up and absorb water.

Flaxseed helps with chronic diarrhea, IBS and other digestive irritations by helping to gently bulk up the stool. The flax mucilage fiber gently cleanses and heals the irritated intestinal tract. Flaxseed fiber will help cleanse the colon and continued usage can help avoid colon cancer.

Complications of Constipation:

- Increase Cholesterol Levels
- Hemorrhoids
- Headaches
- Indigestion
- Varicose veins
- Foul breath
- Body odor
- Indigestion
- May cause increase risk for Colon/ Colorectal/ Rectal cancer
- Diverticulosis

Dose of Flaxseeds - 2-3 tablespoons/day of flaxseed is the general recommendation and can help alleviate and prevent constipation. It is important to drink enough water during/after eating flaxseed, otherwise the colon cannot move the waste material out because the body and colon will compete for the too little amount of water in the body.

Ulcerative Colitis

Ulcerative colitis is a digestive disorder that affects the colon. It often requires dietary changes and the use of regular medications for symptom relief. In some cases, ulcerative colitis may be treated with alternative remedies, such as flaxseed.

It causes inflammation in the linings of the colon and the rectum. As its name implies, ulcerative colitis can also lead to painful ulcers and sores in this lining tissue, usually where cell death has occurred. The sores and inflammation can cause a number of digestive disturbances, including bleeding and frequent, loose stools. Most people's symptoms are mild, however, some people may experience more severe symptoms that involve other bodily systems. Ulcerative colitis can lead to weight loss, joint pain, liver disease and disorders of the eyes. According to the California Pacific Medical Center, both flax seeds and flaxseed oil have been used, along with other dietary supplements, for ulcerative colitis treatment.

Journey of Fiber through food canal

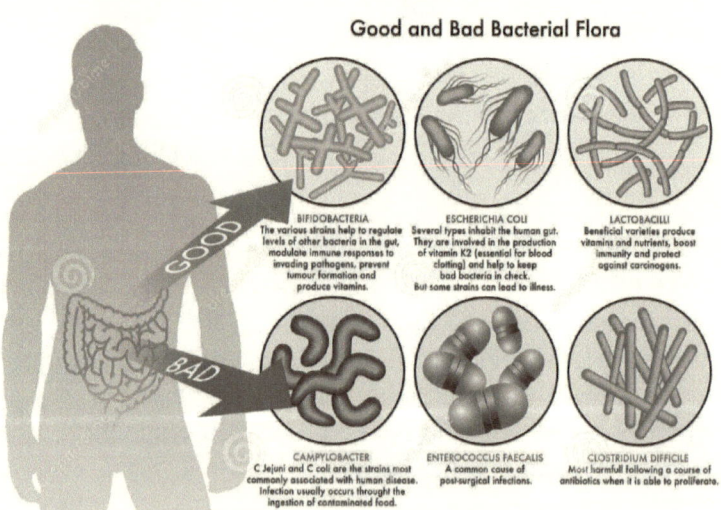

Good and Bad Bacterial Flora

The stomach: In the stomach, as fiber is bulky, so it tends to make us feel full. However, insoluble fiber moves out of the stomach fast unless there is fat, protein, or soluble fiber to slow it down. Soluble fiber, especially the viscous types that absorbs water and swells, will slow down emptying of stomach, especially when eaten with lots of fluid and some fat. This is at least partly why soluble fiber tends to decrease the glycemic effect of a meal - the contents of the stomach more gradually enter the small intestine and from there into the blood.

The small intestine: In the small intestine, it's a similar situation - the presence of insoluble fiber tends to speed up the "transit time", and the gel-like soluble fiber slows things down.

Life in the Colon

It's common thinking that the colon is a place where water is removed from digested food, and the rest is moved along towards the anal opening. But colon does much more for digestion. There is actually a whole world of live bacteria in our guts. There is a huge population of tiny bacteria, roughly ten times as the numbers of all of our human cells (this includes all bacteria from the mouth to the anus). We cannot stay alive without these wonderful friendly creatures in our digestive systems, where battles are fought, helpful substances are produced, vitamins are manufactured, and the immune system is strengthened. In this Disney Land of tiny creatures "The Colon World", the following actions are taken place:

- Vitamins are manufactured (particularly Vitamin K and some B vitamins)
- More minerals are absorbed into the blood
- Friendly bacteria kill the harmful and disease causing bacteria, such as Salmonella
- Friendly bacteria reduce the levels of some toxins
- Some wonderful fats, called short-chain fatty acids, are manufactured, most of which are absorbed into the blood, but some are used as food for the cells of the colon.
- The health of fast growing colon cells, is for the most part dependent upon the tiny bacteria of "Colon World", which in turn is dependent upon the food we provide to these bacteria.

It is the short-chain fatty acids which are getting the most attention recently. It is difficult to get these in our food, so the body relies on the process going on in "Colon World" to make these fats for us. Evidence is building that they are important in keeping the cells of the colon healthy and preventing such conditions as ulcerative colitis, colon cancer, and diverticular disease. They may also help regulate cholesterol and also, to some extent, insulin responses.

Flaxseed and the Immune System

First and most important factor for immune system is alpha-linolenic acid (ALA), an essential omega-3 fatty acid and flaxseed is the richest source of this ALA. Flaxseed contains lignans, a type of phytoestrogen that is also very important for immune system. Recent research suggests that ALA and lignans modulate the immune response and may play a beneficial role in the clinical management of allergic disorders and autoimmune diseases.

Flaxseed Effects on the Immune System

The ALA component of flaxseed influences Immunity - the body's ability to defend itself successfully against foreign invaders - through its effects on membrane phospholipids and the production of eicosanoids and cytokines. Lignans influence certain mediators of the immune response.

Membrane Phospholipids

ALA and other omega-3 fatty acids act by altering the fatty acid composition of membrane phospholipids, which in turn affects eicosanoid production. ALA in flaxseed increases ALA, EPA and DHA levels in phospholipids of mononuclear cells (Lymphocytes), neutrophils and platelets. This change in membrane phospholipid content results in reduced biosynthesis of arachidonic acid from linoleic acid and decreased production of the proinflammatory eicosanoids, leukotriene B4 (LTB4) and thromboxane A2 (TXA2). Increasing the ALA and omega-3 fatty acid content of membrane phospholipids enhances the biosynthesis of anti-inflammatory prostaglandin I3 (PGI3) and other eicosanoids of the 3- and 5-series.

Eicosanoid Production

Pro-inflammatory Eicosanoids

Mediator	Inflammatory Action
Platelet- activating Factor Vasoconstriction (a lipid mediator)	Vasoconstriction PMN[b] activation Increases vascular permeability Platelet aggregation
Prostaglandin (an eicosanoid)	Vasodilatation PMN activation Produces general inflammatory responses such as pain, edema and fever
Thromboxane A2 (an eicosanoid)	Vasoconstriction PMN and platelet activation Stimulates leukocyte adhesion to the endothelium

Eicosanoids are a group of biologically active compounds derived from polyunsaturated fatty acids such as arachidonic acid. In humans, prostaglandin biosynthesis is also influenced by ALA intake. Metabolism of AA by Lipoxygenases (5LOX) result in the production of Leukotrienes E4 and by Thromboxane synthase result in Thromboxane (TXA2)

Cytokine Production

Cytokynes

Mediator	Inflammatory Action
Interleukin 1B	Increases adhesion of molecules to vascular endothelium Stimulates release of other cytokines Induces hepatocytes to produce acute-phase proteins
Interleukin – 6	Activates neutrophils
Tumor necrosis factor	Amplifies inflammatory responses Increases prostaglandin Synthesis Augments fever

Cytokines are soluble proteins liberated from immune cells in response to injury, infection or exposure to foreign substances. Two cytokines that contribute to inflammation are tumor necrosis factor (TNF) and interleukin-1 (IL-1). Both are present in rheumatoid joints and contribute to the tissue pathology of rheumatoid arthritis; and they stimulate the release of platelet-activating factor, a potent mediator of inflammation. The production of TNF and IL-1 by macrophages is influenced by dietary ALA and the ALA to linoleic acid LA ratio. Consumption of a flaxseed-oil based diet for eight weeks, has resulted in an inhibition of TNF and IL-1 b production of about 77-81% in a study of 28 healthy men.

Uses of Flaxseed in autoimmune diseases

Flaxseed favorably influences immune response. The flaxseed ALA, alters membrane phospholipids, inhibits arachidonic acid biosynthesis from linoleic acid, inhibits the production of pro-inflammatory eicosanoids from arachidonic acid, and suppresses lymphocyte proliferation and cytokine production. Flaxseed lignans are potent inhibitors of platelet-activating factor, a mediator of inflammation. Through these effects, flaxseed has the potential to be used for the treatment of disorders characterized in part by activated lymphocytes and a hyper-stimulated immune response. Such disorders include rheumatoid arthritis, psoriasis, multiple sclerosis, systemic lupus erythematosus and other allergic disorders.

Atherosclerosis and Flaxseeds

Flaxseed inhibits the production of major systemic markers of inflammation, including eicosanoids, cytokines and platelet-activating factor. Regular consumption of flaxseed may interfere with the progression of atherosclerosis, an inflammatory disease. Atherosclerosis is an inflammatory disease. Its

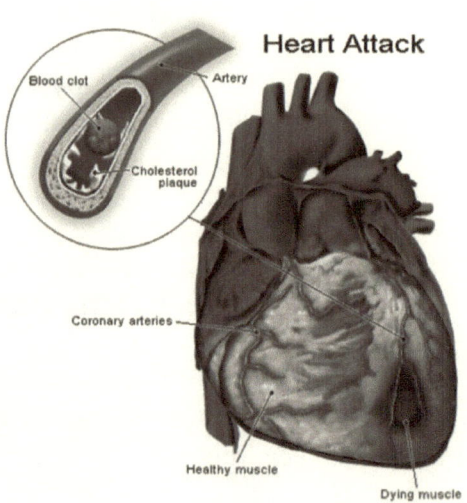

origins are in infancy and childhood when the earliest lesions, called fatty streaks, begin to develop in arteries. These fatty streaks consist only of monocyte derived macrophages and T lymphocytes - two types of immune cells, whose presence in arterial walls provides evidence that the inflammation contributes to atherosclerosis. After understanding the role of inflammation in atherosclerosis, scientists develop a new dimension to cardiovascular disease prevention and treatment by developing therapies that alleviate chronic inflammation, may retard the progression of atherosclerosis.

Atherosclerosis and the Inflammatory Response

The earliest changes in Atherosclerosis occur in the arterial endothelium. The endothelium becomes more permeable to lipoproteins and immune system cells such as monocytes, T lymphocytes and leukocytes. The migration of these immune cells into arterial walls is mediated by oxidized low-density lipoprotein (LDL), cytokines and other blood factors. Cytokines are proteins synthesized and released by macrophages, leukocytes, neutrophils and other cells; they initiate and amplify inflammatory responses. Fatty streaks consisting of lipid and cholesterol-rich monocytes, macrophages and T lymphocytes begin to form in arteries. This process is stimulated by the adherence and aggregation of platelets and by several mediators of the inflammatory response, including growth factors, cytokines such as interleukin-1 and tumor necrosis factor, and thromboxane A2, an eicosanoid derived from arachidonic acid.

With continued inflammation, the fatty streaks progress to advanced, complicated lipid-filled lesions. Eventually, a fibrous cap forms. Formation of the fibrous cap represents a healing response to the injury and is mediated by the actions of interleukin-1, tumor necrosis factor and other cytokines. When the advanced lesion becomes unstable, the plaque ruptures, causing a thrombosis that may result in myocardial infarction or stroke.

How Flaxseed benefits in Atherosclerosis

Flaxseed reduces inflammatory activity. This effect is likely due to one or both of the following constituents present in flaxseed: alpha-linolenic acid (ALA), the essential omega-3 fatty, and lignans, that exhibit antioxidant, anti-inflammatory and anti-fungal activity. Flaxseed is the richest source of ALA with its unique fatty acid profile. ALA constitutes 57% of the total fatty acids in flaxseed.

ALA and the other omega-3 fatty acids block the conversion of linoleic acid, an essential omega-6 fatty acid, to arachidonic acid and they inhibit the synthesis of pro-inflammatory eicosanoids, such as thromboxane A2 derived from arachidonic acid. Flaxseed also inhibits the release of several inflammatory cytokines—namely, tumor necrosis factor (TNF-a), interleukin-1ß (IL-1ß) and interleukin-6 (IL-6). ALA is itself converted to the long-chain fatty acid eicosapentaenoic acid (EPA). EPA is converted to eicosanoids that are less biologically active than those derived from arachidonic acid and hence do not promote inflammation and platelet aggregation.

Flaxseed lignans are PAF-receptor antagonists and thus block the pro-inflammatory actions of PAF (PAF is a biologically active compound that is derived from arachidonic acid and is involved in many immunopathological reactions.). Furthermore, lignans may act like other antioxidants in blocking the oxidation of LDL particles and decreasing their deposition in arterial walls. The oxidation of LDL is believed to be a key pathological event in the development of atherosclerosis.

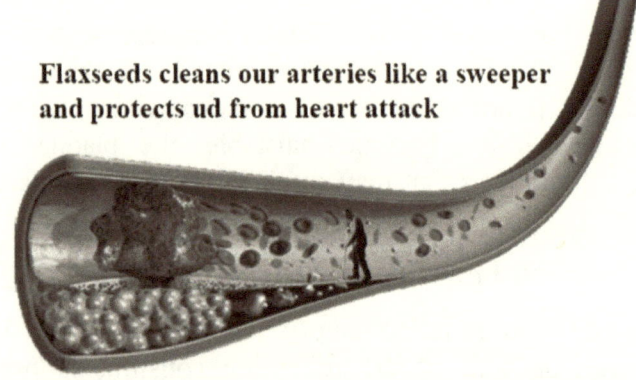

Flaxseeds cleans our arteries like a sweeper and protects ud from heart attack

Flax Lowers Cholesterol and May Have Long-term Benefits on Heart

Eating 2-6 tbsp (15-50 g) of milled flax daily for as little as 4 weeks decreased blood total and LDL-cholesterol significantly in clinical studies. (LDL-cholesterol is the so-called bad cholesterol.) Blood total cholesterol decreased 6-13% and LDL-cholesterol decreased 9-18% in studies of healthy young adults, 5,6 men and women with moderately high levels of blood cholesterol, and other groups. HDL cholesterol (the so-called good cholesterol) and triglycerides did not change in these studies.

The beneficial effect of milled flax and whole flax seeds may be due in part to the dietary fiber in flax. Flax contains mucilage gums, which are a type of soluble dietary fiber. Soluble dietary fiber helps lower blood cholesterol levels. In a study of 29 adults with high blood cholesterol levels, blood total cholesterol decreased about 5.5% and LDL-cholesterol decreased 9.7% when the volunteers ate muffins made with partially defatted flax for 3 weeks compared with when they ate muffins made from wheat bran for 3 weeks. (Partially defatted flax contains less than 10% fat, compared with regular milled flax, which contains about 41% fat.) These findings suggest a role for flax mucilage gums in lowering blood lipids.

A regular intake of flaxseed may help treat coronary heart disease and stroke by reducing blood cholesterol levels, and it may help retard the progression of atherosclerosis by reducing inflammatory responses.

Flaxseed protect fatal Arrhythmias

Arrhythmias are abnormal rhythms of the heart muscle. There are many different types of arrhythmias. Some are insignificant because they cause the heart muscle to skip a beat or add an extra beat, and they are not dangerous. Others are serious, resulting in dizzy spells, shortness of breath, chest pain and other complications. The large number of sudden cardiac deaths from coronary heart disease – estimated at about 8-10% of all deaths in Canada in 1999 and 335,000 deaths per year in the United States – are due mainly to arrhythmia.

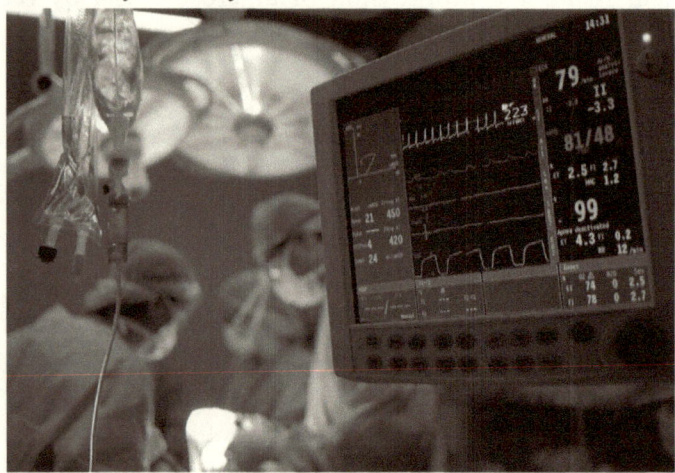

Growing evidence suggests a simple dietary change – increasing the dietary intake of omega-3 fats – may help prevent sudden death from arrhythmias. The major omega-3 fats are alpha-linolenic acid (ALA), the essential omega-3 fatty acid, and its long-chain cousins, eicosapentaenoic acid (EPA) and docosahexaenoic acid (DHA).

The omega-3 fatty acids prevent arrhythmias in heart cells grown in test tubes and also in laboratory animals. In humans, omega-3 fats have been shown to reduce the risk of arrhythmias in most, but not all, clinical studies.

How Arrhythmias Occur in the Heart

The heart is a duplex four room apartment that pumps blood throughout the body. The pumping action of the heart is controlled by electrical signals, which are produced by a special group of cells located in the heart's right upper room. These special cells are known collectively as the sinus node. The sinus node is a electricity generator for the heart. Its electrical signals travel first through the upper rooms of the heart (the atria), then through a switching relay called the AV node, and finally to the lower rooms of the heart (the ventricles). The ventricles route the electrical signal through special nerve cells, and the end result is a contraction of the heart muscle, which pumps blood through the body. Arrhythmias occur when the heart's natural generator, the sinus node, develops an unnatural rhythm. In some cases, the sinus node may beat too fast, producing a condition known as tachycardia. In other cases, the sinus node's electrical signal is totally disorganized, causing the atria to contract too quickly. Both conditions are very serious.

Omega-3 Fats Protect against Arrhythmia in Test Tube Studies

Omega-3 fats may protect against arrhythmia by helping heart muscle cells remain stable electrically and by preventing them from becoming "hyper excitable". In test tube studies of rat heart cells, for example, omega-3 fats decreased the electrical excitability of the heart cells, making them less likely to develop abnormal heart rhythms.

The omega-3 fats worked by blocking the entry of calcium into the heart muscle cells. DHA and ALA were better than EPA at blocking calcium entry into these cells. (Calcium works like a pacemaker for cells, much like the sinus node is a pacemaker for the heart.) These findings suggest that the anti-arrhythmic effect of omega-3 fats is partly due to their ability to control the electrical activity of cells.

Alpha-Linolenic Acid Is As Effective as EPA and DHA in Animals

Pure preparations of ALA, EPA and DHA are equally good at protecting against fatal arrhythmias in dogs. In one study, pure solutions of ALA, EPA and DHA were infused separately. All three omega-3 fats reduced significantly the occurrence of ventricular fibrillation and protected a majority of dogs from fatal arrhythmias. Infusion of a control fat (soybean oil) failed to protect any animals from fatal arrhythmias. These findings suggest that omega-3 fats help regulate heart function.

What is diabetes?

Diabetes is a defect in the body's ability to convert glucose (sugar) to energy. Glucose is the main source of fuel for our body. When food is digested it is changed into fats, protein, or carbohydrates. Foods that affect blood sugars are called carbohydrates. Carbohydrates, when digested, change to glucose. Examples of some carbohydrates are: bread, rice, pasta, potatoes, corn, fruit, and milk products. Individuals with diabetes may eat carbohydrates but must do so in moderation.

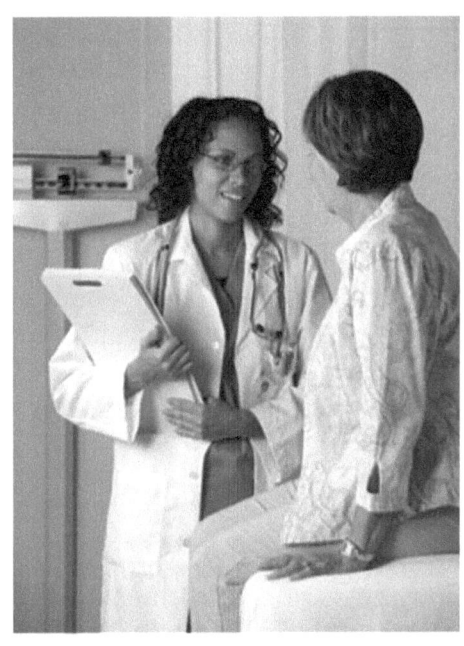

Glucose is then transferred into the blood and is used by the cells for energy. In order for glucose to be transferred from the blood to the cells, the hormone - insulin is needed. Insulin is produced by the beta cells in the pancreas.

Chronic Inflammation is Cause of Type 2 Diabetes

Researchers at the University of California, San Diego School of Medicine have discovered that chronic inflammation provoked by immune cells called macrophages leads to insulin resistance and Type 2 diabetes.

Dr. Budwig had written in her book that Diabetes is basically a Fat syndrome (a disorder of Fat Metabolism), the sugar problem is secondary and comes later into the picture.

Preventing Diabetes by daily Flaxseed consumption

ADA 2011 LIVE/71st Scientific Session 24-28th June 2011/San Diego, California.

Flaxseed is a good source of Omega-3 Fatty acids and viscous fiber. Consuming flaxseed on regular basis may reduce the risk of progressing from pre-diabetes to type 2 diabetes and heart disease through various mechanisms. One recent study has shown that 13-26 g. of flaxseed daily in addition to regular diet, can decrease glucose, insulin and insulin sensitivity in individuals with pre-diabetes.

Clinical ADAA Randomized, controlled study presented during session: Nutrition Clinical Author: Andrea Hutchins, Blakely Y D.Brown, Stethane Domitrowich, Earle Adams, Courtney Bobowies: Colorado Springs, CO, Missoula.

Courtesy - Dr. N.K.Singh , DHRC, Dhanbad http://www.dhrcindia.com

Flax for Diabetes

Flaxseed - a nutritional powerhouse whole grain food has so many benefits for fighting diabetes. As part of a balanced and healthy diet, flax is so excellent because it helps stabilize blood sugar and controls/prevents diabetes.

Flax is a low glycemic food and has many benefits due to the Omega 3, fiber, protein and lignans found in flaxseed.

Our body's operating system performs high tech multi tasking operations. Sugar and insulin are very important. When we eat food, our body produces insulin to help keep blood sugar levels under control. The more vegetables, whole grains and low glycemic foods we eat, the easier it is for our body to keep blood sugars stable and within the normal levels.

The more processed foods, sugar, white flours, white rice, etc we eat the harder it will be to control blood sugar levels and the more likely it is that we will suffer from diabetes and its consequences.

Flax seed - low glycemic zero carb food

Flaxseed is an excellent low glycaemic food (G.I. of flax is 32) and it helps stabilize blood sugars. This means that blood sugar levels that spike when you eat sugary and white flour/ white rice type of foods will not spike when you eat flax.

With flax, blood sugar levels will slowly and smoothly rise to a lower curve and then the blood sugar levels will stay there for a longer period of time. After a few hours, your blood sugar level will slowly go down, this is the key to how flaxseed benefits diabetes.

How flax is Zero carb – sweet mathematics

Flaxseed is a Zero Carb food; let me explain this with just simple mathematics?

14 Gm of Flaxseed contains		
	Protein	2.56 gm,
	Fat	5.9 gm,
	Moisture	0.97 gm
	Ash	0.53 gm
Total is 0.97+2.56+5.90+0.53 =		9.86 gm.

In these 4.04 gms of carb Flax has got 3.8 gm fiber, **So actual sugar is 4.04 – 3.8 = 0.24 gm**, which is comparatively negligible amount so practically Flax is called a **ZERO** carb food.

(Remember fiber belongs to carbs but is not absorbed in the intestines and does not raise blood sugar level)

Fiber keeps sugar absorption slow and steady

Flax has 3 fibers insoluble, soluble and mucilage fiber (a type of soluble fiber). These fibers fill up the stomach and take longer to digest - this means that blood sugar level spikes slowly, remains steady for longer and so we feel full for longer!

Our blood sugars don't have to constantly fluctuate up and down because the fiber keeps them stable for longer. Soluble fiber slows down the absorption of glucose and helps the body manage glucose levels and insulin production smoothly.

Flax for diabetics is an economical and powerful step to help stabilize blood sugars toward the goals of fighting and preventing diabetes!

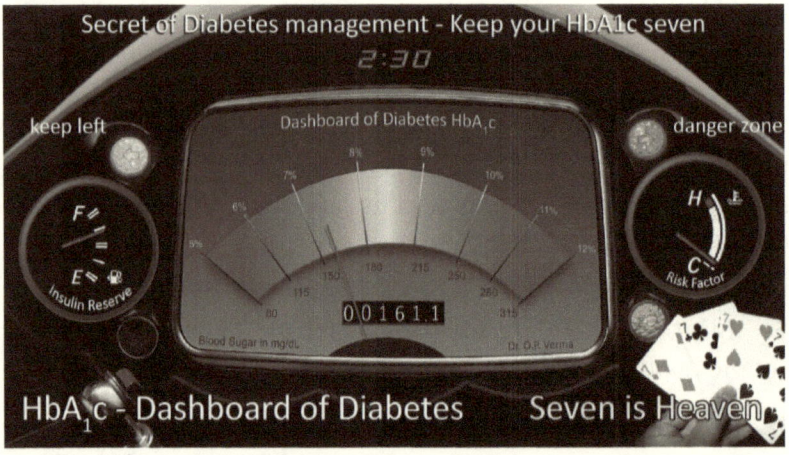

Omega-3 – Helps Your Brain feel Satiated & helps stop food cravings!

Most of us are not getting enough Omega 3 in our diet. This is a problem because Omega 3 is essential and our bodies cannot make its own omega-3 - our body must get this from what we eat.

One of the important roles of omega 3 is to tell our brains that we are full and satiated. When we aren't eating enough omega 3, our brain thinks that we are hungry and our body is craving for the nutrition, which it needs. A great way to take a small step toward health is adding flaxseed so that diabetes can be better controlled or prevented.

Omega-3 helps prevents Chronic Inflammation

Diabetes results from chronic inflammation. This means in diabetes our body is constantly burning at a low fire. Blood vessels become hard, brittle and narrow, insulation of nerves are damaged, body doesn't function properly and cellular aging is enhanced. This leads to many complications.

Omega-3 fatty acids produce anti-inflammatory, anti-clotting (thrombolytic), vasodilatory prostaglandins, cytokines and leukotrines. Thus Not only can flaxseed help stabilize blood sugar levels for longer periods of time, but it can also help the body heal and prevent worsening diabetes along with complications that many diabetics presently suffer from or could potentially have later on.

Flax lignans – stabilize blood sugar levels

Lignans help to heal the body, including the pancreas, which is a key player in how the body manages Insulin. Thus Lignans stabilize blood sugar levels. Lignans are powerful antioxidants and prevents aging.

Flax – prevents and cures complications

Heart –

- Flax lowers blood pressure.
- Flax lowers triglycerides, total and LDL Cholesterol. It also raises HDL cholesterol.
- Flax is a natural aspirin – flax acts as a blood thinner by so interfering with platelets' ability to stick together.
- Regular flax eaters don't need any aspirin or statin.
- Flax prevents fatal arrhythmia.
- Flax is powerful antioxidant and anti-inflammatory.

Foot –

- Flax enhances proper blood circulation in foot and reverses nerve damage, thus prevents peripheral neuropathy and trophic ulcers.
- Flax keeps skin and foot healthy.
- Flax prevents infections, ulcers, wounds, gangrene as well as amputations.

Sexual insufficiency –

- Again due to vascular and nerve damage diabetic patient develops sexual problems.
- Flax prevents and cures Sexual problems of male as well as females.

Eye –

- Due to blood vessel damage patient develop diabetic Retinopathy, which ultimately causes blindness. Flax keeps blood vessels healthy and ensures better circulation so it prevents Retinopathy.
- Flax delays cataract and prevents glaucoma.
- Flaxseed oil is best lubricant eye drops and helps in dry eye syndrome.

No refined oil

Refined vegetable oils have been stripped of most of their nutritional value, while Natural oils contain vitamins, minerals and other nutritional factors. The process of extracting the oils destroys this nutritive value. Refined oils are usually extracted using heat, then degummed. They are usually partially hydrogenated, a process which involves adding hydrogen to the oil in the presence of nickel.

The final stage of making refined oil is to bleach it. Sodium hydroxide is added to remove free fatty acids and the bleaching process also removes beta-carotene and the essential oils.

No trans fat

Processed oils are often heated to high temperatures, a process which causes the formation of trans-fats. Heating oils to just 300 degrees starts the process of causing fatty acids to become mutagenic (cancer causing). Trans-fatty acids start forming at 320 degrees and at 392 degrees significant quantities of trans-fats are formed. The more you reuse an oil for frying, the more trans fats you'll create.

For deep frying use coconut oil. This medium-chain saturated fat is very heat stable and is also good for you. Butter, clarified butter and olive oil are at least better than hydrogenated fats for deep frying. Water is best medium for frying. For light stir frying mustard oil is right choice.

How to incorporate flax in your diet

Ideally, flax seed should be consumed in the grounded form or as its oil. Remember that flax seed oil does not contains the fiber or lignans etc.

Flax Bread or Chapatti - The best way to mix freshly ground flaxseed with multigrain flour and makes chapatti, bread or pancake. **In diabetes ideally take 20 gms flaxseed twice daily.**

Start slowly if you aren't used to a high-fiber diet. Grind it coarsely and drink plenty of water. You could have it with your cereals, yogurt or milk, shakes and smoothies or even add it to homemade cookies, vegetables or salads.

To get maximum benefits, 30 to 50 grams of ground flax is recommended per day.

In short, this is how flaxseed terminates diabetes?

- Zero Carb Food
- Hypoglycemia
- Anti-inflammatory
- Increase BMR & eliminates food craving
- Anti-obesity
- Anti-Platelet
- Anti-hypertensive
- Anti-arrhythmic
- Anti-thrombotic
- Anti-atherogenic
- Improves Endothelial Function
- Anti-cholesterol
- Coronary Vasodilator

- Improves Heart Risk Parameters
- Improves Vision Color Fidelity
- Delays cataract and reduces intraocular Pressure
- Peripheral Vasodilator
- Natural Cosmetic
- Natural Manicure and Pedicure
- Rejuvenates Nerves and Brain cells
- Anti-lupus
- Anti-depressant
- Mood Elevator - A Feel Good Food
- Nootropic - Enhances Memory & Cognition
- Aphrodisiac - Cures Sexual Problems

Some Natural Remedies for Diabetes

Colostrum - So how could colostrum able to benefit all 3 types of diabetic conditions? In the nutshell, colostrum contains 'Low Molecular Weight Chromium-binding peptide' and research shown it increases the receptors of insulin on the surface of the cells in the body. These receptors increase the uptake of insulin and therefore may reduce the sugar in the blood. This helps those with insulin resistance condition (type 2 diabetes), including pregnant women experiencing gestational diabetes.

Also found in colostrum is a type of peptide call 'obestatin'. Research done so far on mice shown that this peptide could prevent the death of insulin-producing beta cells in the pancreas and also increases the beta cell population in the pancreas. It is well-known that colostrum contains immunomodulatory properties which could calm an over-active immune function. So as colostrum reduces the effect of the autoimmune effects destroying the beta cells in the pancreas, the 'obestatin' on the other hand, is helping to repopulated the insulin-producing beta cells in the pancreas.

Magnesium - Although the relationship between magnesium and diabetes has been studied for decades, it is not yet fully understood. Studies show that a deficiency in magnesium may worsen blood sugar control in type 2 diabetes. Scientists say that a deficiency of magnesium interrupts insulin secretion in the pancreas and increases insulin resistance in the body's tissues. Evidence suggests that a deficiency of magnesium may contribute to certain diabetes complications.

Vanadium - Vanadium is a compound found in tiny amounts in plants and animals. Early studies showed that vanadium normalized blood sugar levels in animals with type 1 and type 2 diabetes. A recent study found that when people with diabetes were given vanadium, they developed a modest increase in insulin sensitivity and were able to decrease their insulin requirements. The richest source of Vanadium is radish.

Black Seed - Black seed, also known as Nigella Sativa is a cure for all diseases, except death and considered to be a miraculous cure. For seven days take 6 teaspoons of the oil. Take the oil three different times of the day. Then take 2 teaspoons in the morning and 2 in the evening for 4 days. Follow by taking 2 teaspoons of the oil for two days. Take plenty of water in the morning and rub the oil all over the body for 10 days. You must mix the oil with fruit juice. Repeat this treatment if you do not see any improvement.

Cinnamon - Cinnamon has long been reported as a good source for the treatment of diabetes, due to a study done in 2003 by Khan and associates. 60 people were tested in the group and one third of the group was given a placebo. The end results were very impressive and the overall health of the group was increased with glucose down 18 percent; LDL cholesterol and triglycerides also showed reduced levels. Everyone was excited and the word of using cinnamon spread.

Bitter Melon - Researchers have proven that bitter melon works great with the treatment of diabetes. It contains insulin like properties which help in the lowering of the blood and urine levels. It is suggested to be used frequently. The bitter melon should be juiced and then taken on an empty stomach before eating first thing in the morning. The seeds may be ground to a powder and eaten also. You can also, make a tea from the bitter melon.

Science of Memory

Memory is an internal mental storage that we maintain, which give us instant access to our personal past, complete with all of the facts that we know and the skills that we have achieved. The following are primary stages of the human memory process.

- **Encoding**
- **Storage**
- **Retrieval**
- **Forgetting** may constitute the fourth stage of memory, although forgetting is technically a failure in memory retrieval.

During the **encoding stage**, information is sent to brain, where it is processed and composed into most appropriate manner. Some specialized brain cells analyze incoming stimuli and compose that information into a specialized neural code. In the **storage stage** of memory formation, the brain must retain encoded data over extended periods of time. **Retrieval stage** brings out the permanent memory back into working memory, which can be mentally manipulated for current usage.

Science of Memory

Learning is an active process that involves sensory input into the brain, which occurs automatically, and an ability to extract meaningful information from sensory input. Then storing that information into working (short-term) memory, where consideration for transfer into permanent (long-term) memory takes place.

Vision has a much longer impact in the human memory than does the printed word. By exploiting this competency, students learn quickly when they can visualize the concept while studying, by directed use of the mind's eye, where mental pictures can be developed.

Writing words in the air on an imaginary blackboard forces students not only to visualize the order of letters in a word, but to maintain visually what they have already written in working memory as they continue to write. When young learners are taught to construct diagrams that show relationships, their memory of content improves substantially.

Once the elements that make up an experience are classified according to their special traits, each part is shunted to a different brain region for further detailed analysis. The various pieces of new information get stored in neural circuits distributed throughout the cerebral cortex. Because the elements making up a memory reside in multiple cortical areas, the stronger the network linking the associated pieces together, the more resistant to it will be to forgetting.

As the brain transacts learning events, physical changes occur both within brain circuitry and in its structure-function correlations. Memory is quite liquid, and, over time, the brain continues to revisit and reorganize stored information with each subsequent experience, reprogramming its contents through a repetitive updating procedure known as brain plasticity. This is advantageous, since improvements are made repeatedly to existing data. Prior knowledge is revised based on new input, resulting in a more accurate representation of the current world, increasing one's probability of thriving.

Memory decay

While memory cannot occur without learning, once information has been learned, our memory may allow the learning to decay. Stress and multitasking are among the chief causes of memory lapses. Memory failure most likely reflects the consequences of stress, poor nutrition and exhaustion.

Emotions

Emotions can be a catalyst to learning. In school, mere exposure to content information (lecture, text, etc.) is no guarantee that it will reach the personal/emotional threshold of the learner, where encoding the information for permanent memory storage is deemed warranted. What students encode depends on what they are paying attention to at the time.

Hippocmpus – The Site for Memory Building

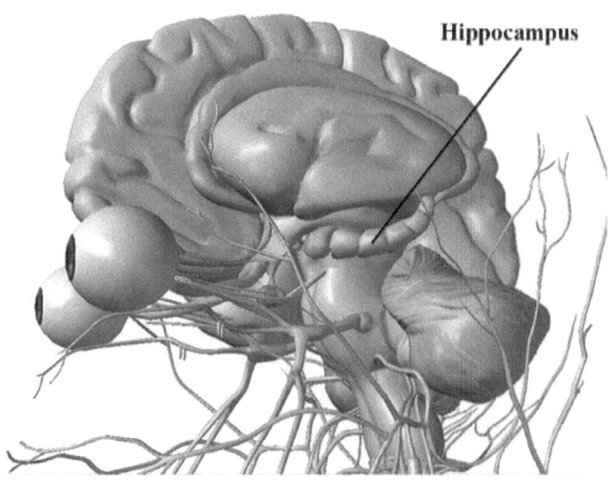

Several connected brain regions play key roles in memory formation, including the thalamus, amygdala, hippocampus and cerebral cortex. It is the interaction of nearly all parts of the brain that allows for the construction of our memories.

The hippocampus plays a crucial role in forming and storing our memories of facts and events. Initially, short-term memories are briefly stored in the hippocampus, prior to being transferred to other brain regions where they are consolidated with prior knowledge into long-term memories. As Stanford Ericksen summarized the requisite emotional element in learning, "Students learn what they care about and remember what they understand."

When information is determined to have potential long-term value, the hippocampus links the significant elements of that event or experience together, forming a permanent memory. Brain-imaging studies have shown heightened activations in the hippocampus when we are recalling memories. This has important implications concerning creativity and innovation, which are based on our ability to manipulate and expand on stored factual information.

Emotional experiences (both positive and negative) enjoy the highest probability of reaching permanent memory storage. It is the amygdala-hippocampus connection that fosters the development of our most memorable moments in life. In the classroom, emotions determine what students pay attention to, which impacts what students will later remember.

When attempting to memorize unrelated terms, mnemonics present the most practical solution. For students attempting to remember the most important neurotransmitters, the term "San Dope" works effectively.

- Serotonin 5-Hydroxytryptamine
- Acetylcholine
- Norepinephrine
- Dopamine
- Oxytocin
- Phenylethanolamine
- Epinephrine (adrenaline)

Omega-3 increase membrane fluidity

The brain has a huge number of cell membranes are made out of fat. The fat content of the brain is a little different than the rest of the body - only PUFAs allowed into the healthy brain in any appreciable amount are the ALA omega 3 derived DHA (a long-chain omega 3 fatty acid) and the LA omega 6 derived arachidonic acid (AA). In addition, while AA is found in equal amounts all over the brain, DHA is found predominately in the gray matter. That's where our thinking takes place.

Let me explain a bit about the actual structure of these molecules. Saturated fats make rather tough and hard cell membranes all on their own. Their structure is pretty straight and tough, and they make cell membranes that look like this:

Iiiiiiiiiiiiiiiiiiiiiiiiiiiiiiiiiiiiiiiiiiiiiiiiiiiiiiiiiiiiiiiiii

PUFAs have unsaturated double bonds, which make them bend and become weaker at double bonds. cell membrane made of PUFAs that look like this:

iiiiiLiiiiiiiiiiLiiiiiiiiiLiiiiiLiiiiiiiiiiiiiLiiiiiiii

You can see that the unsaturated double bonds break up the structure a bit, and Dr. Paul Jaminet call this "increasing membrane fluidity." Important cell membrane proteins, such as ion channels, depend on the presence of PUFAs to be incorporated correctly into the membrane. If all is well, the PUFAs serve as part of "lipid rafts" that are required for transport of protein and signals through the membranes, the formation of synapses, and maintaining the integrity of the neuronal membranes. All of these functions are dependent upon omega-3 fats and are important and vital for the brilliant functioning of our complex brains.

Dr. Paul had nicely represented the role of PUFAs in neuronal cell membranes by simple "L" and "i" drawing of the cell membrane:

Omega 3 fats - especially DHA - are unique mainly in that they don't possess any real shape. They have so many double bonds that can twist and bend so easily, they change the shape very rapidly and under the slightest pressure fold up into tiny balls or slip out of the way. This is what makes salmon oil so slippery, especially at body temperature.

So a omega-3 rich membrane is barely a membrane at all. Rather a unique soap bubble like structure. A biological extreme. We don't even have a suitable letter in the alphabets for it; even M has only three bends. DHA has six double bonds. This is what human intelligent brain depends on.

We can make sufficient DHA from ALA omega 3 found in flaxseed, if we have niacin, vitamin B-6, vitamin-C, magnesium and zinc in our body. We have enough evidence that if you consume flaxseeds regularly, your body makes sufficient DHA required for high end brain.

The omega 6 derived AA is also important in the brain - it initiates and controls the inflammatory response, which is a critical function. The ratio of omega-3 and omega-6 is also very important, most ideal being 1:4. We can also make sufficient AA from LA omega 6 found in flaxseed, if we have niacin, vitamin B-6, vitamin-C, magnesium and zinc in our body.

Omega-3 Fats- Reversing Many Aspects of Neurologic Aging

The cardio protective power of omega-3 fatty acids has been thoroughly understood in clinical literature. Less well known is their paramount role in optimizing many facets of brain function, from depression to cognition and from memory to mental health.

Recent research has opened up a new horizon in our understanding of omega-3s' profound ability to recover age-related decline and breaking the long-held medical belief that brain shrinkage and nerve cell death is progressive and irreversible. Omega-3s have been shown to have antidepressant and neuroprotective properties.

Omega-3 - Key Nutrient from the Cradle to the Grave

Approximately 30% of the brain's dry weight is omega-3 fatty acids - the building block for an estimated 100 billion neurons. They play a host of vital roles in neuronal structure and function, protecting them from oxidative damage, inflammation, and the cumulative destruction imposed by other chronic insults.

Embedded in the omega-3-rich neuronal membrane are numerous proteins and complex molecules required for electrochemical transmission and signal reception. Scientists have recently shown that the precise balance of fatty acids in brain cells helps determine whether a given nerve cell will be protected against injury or inflammation, or whether it will instead succumb to the injury.

Omega-3s accumulate in the human brain during fetal development. The amount of the omega-3 has been closely tied to intelligence and cognitive performance in infancy and childhood. Early deficits in brain content of omega-3s have been associated with poor brain development and neurocognitive dysfunction. These are manifested especially in the area of attention, increasing the risk for attention-deficit/hyperactivity disorder (ADHD) and other behavioral disturbances. Later in life, declining levels of Omega-3 fats may contribute to development of aggression, anxiety, depression, schizophrenia, dementia, and a variety of other mental health and even criminal conditions.

Scientists are having great success at reversing many of the fundamental age-related decreases in brain function correlated with omega-3 deficiency. ADHD and related conditions can be prevented or corrected by supplementing infants and nursing mothers with Omega-3.   A remarkable animal study has just revealed that omega-3 fatty acids halt the age-related loss of brain cell receptors vital to memory production, and show potential for increasing neuronal growth.

Omega-3 - A Natural Crime Cutter ?

Recent findings suggest that some criminal and aggressive behaviors are closely correlated with low omega-3 levels, which are linked to lower levels of honesty, and self-discipline. These effects may be related to alterations in serotonin turnover, which controls impulsivity and aggression-hostility behaviors.

There's solid data indicating that optimal omega-3 intake at all ages is a promising factor for subsiding aggression and hostility. For example, omega-3 supplementation in autistic children with severe tantrums, aggression, or self-injurious behavior produced significant improvements, without adverse side effects. And stressed but otherwise healthy volunteers given Omega-3 Fats reported a significantly improved rate of stress reduction, suggesting an adaptogenic role for omega-3s (adaptogens help the body respond to imposed stress in a variety of ways).

In a group of drug abusers, supplementation with Omega-3 Fats for 3 months produced significant decreases in anger and anxiety scores compared. Similarly, in young adult prison inmates, multi-supplements featuring omega-3s produced significant reductions in antisocial, violent, aggressive, and transgressive (rule-breaking) behavior.

Omega-3 – Cures Cognitive Decline and Memory Disorders

Omega-3 intake is strongly associated with cognition and memory in numerous studies. Insufficient omega-3 intake is strongly correlated with diminished adaptability of brain synapses and impaired learning and memory. People with lower omega-3 levels may be more likely to suffer from a host of cognitive impairments including dyslexia, ADHD, and cognitive decline.

Laboratory studies throw light on these observations, suggesting that omega-3 supplementation may enhance brain function through increased production of the membrane-rich neurons required for new synapse formation. Other protective and cognition-enhancing effects include improved neuronal cell membrane characteristics resulting in enhanced neurotransmission, increased synaptic release of vital neurotransmitters such as serotonin, and neuroprotection from inflammation and oxidant-related damage including those induced by antipsychotic medications.

In healthy adults, increased omega-3 intake is positively associated with greater brain volume in regions associated with emotional arousal and regulation of behavior. People who get more omega-3s have bigger, more functional brains.

Flaxseed - Sim Card of Mind

Think of your brain like the engine in your car. It needs oil just like your car does. Omega 3 is that oil. It helps things to run smoothly and efficiently. In the function of development of our brain, Omega 3 is vital for memory and performance, and it is needed for the transmission and reception of brain signals. In addition to the structural benefits in the brain that Omega 3 adds, it aids in the communication between brain cells.

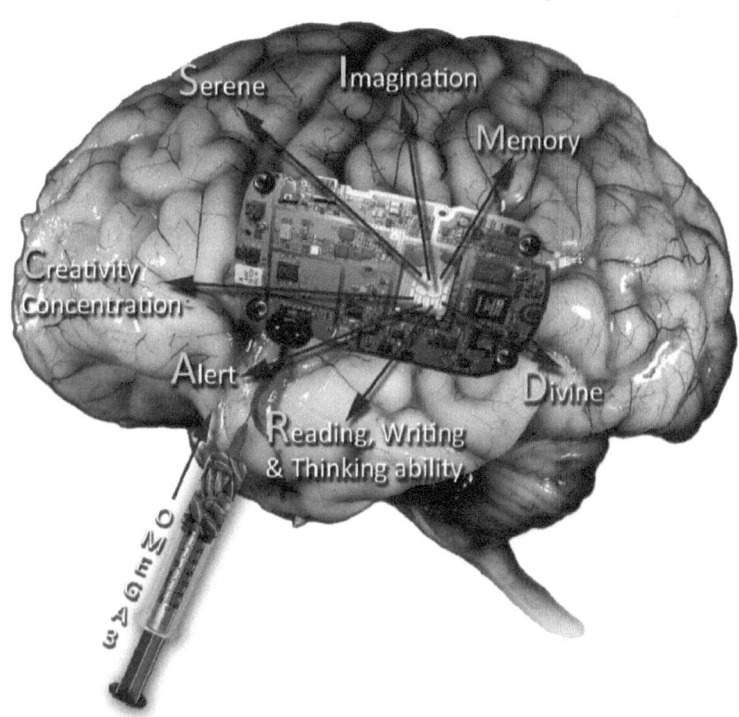

Flaxseed is SIM CARD of mind's circuit (Mnemonic of flaxseed benefits on mind). Here SIM means Serene, Imagination & Memory and CARD denotes Creativity & Concentration, Alertness, Reading writing & thinking ability and divine. Flax has been scientifically proven to treat depression, diabetic neuropathy, ADHD, Alzheimer's disease, Parkinson's disease, multiple sclerosis and proven to improve the behavior of Schizophrenics. Flaxseed can improve eyesight and perception of colors. Colors look bolder and vivid. Life becomes simply more colorful.

Flaxseed - Feel Good Food

The Flaxseed is a feel good food, keeps your mind cool and you stay cheerful. Negative thoughts stay far away from you. You don't become angry. Your mood is always elated and positive. This is super anti-depressant. Flaxseeds are essential for the function and structure of the brain, improve cognition, memory learning skill and concentration.

Budwig Protocol

We are fighting with cancer since the dawn of history. Every year we discover new diagnostic modalities, better radiotherapy techniques and lots of new chemotherapy drugs. But we have completely failed to defeat this disease called cancer. Think again, are we really going on the right path? Does conventional Medicine really attack on the prime cause of cancer???

What is the prime cause of Cancer?

All normal cells absolutely require oxygen, but cancer cells can live without oxygen - a rule without exception. Deprive a cell 35% of its oxygen for 48 hours and it would become cancerous. Dr. Otto Warburg clearly mentioned that the root cause of cancer is lack of oxygen in the cells (Schmid).

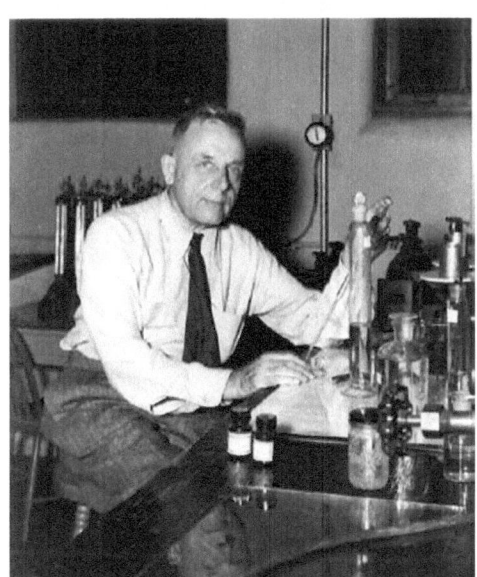

He also discovered that cancer cells are anaerobic (do not breathe oxygen), get the energy by fermenting glucose and produce lactic acid. The body becomes acidic. Cancer cannot survive in the presence of high levels of oxygen, as found in an alkaline state. He got Noble Prize for this great discovery in 1931 (Nobelprize.org).

He postulated that sulfur containing protein and some unknown fat is required to attract oxygen in the cell. This fat plays a major role in the respiration and functioning of Warburg respiratory enzyme. He thought it would be butyric acid and made experiment, but this attempt was a failure. For many decades scientists were trying to identify this unknown and mysterious fat but nobody succeeded.

Dr. Johanna Budwig was a qualified pharmacologist, chemist and physicist with a doctorate in physics who worked as the chief expert for drugs and fats at the Federal Institute for Fats Research, Germany. She was known as a leading authority on fats and oils in the world.

In 1949, Dr. Budwig developed new ways of testing fats through the development of Paper Chromatography. This meant that for the first time fats, fatty acids and lipoproteides could be detected directly even in the smallest proportions and 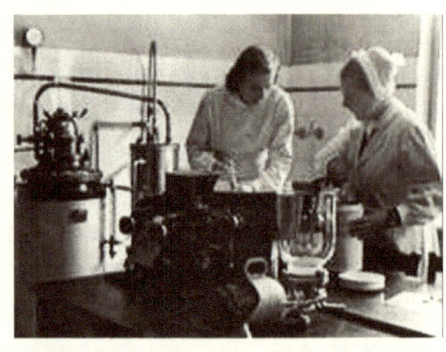 thus characterized and studied in the form of microanalysis. Using Cobalt 60 isotopes she was successful in producing the first differentiation reaction to identify fatty acids, and via radioiodine produced the first direct iodine value. She also developed control of atmosphere in closed system by using gas systems which act as antioxidants. Coloring, separating effects of fats and fatty acids were further developed. Behavior of fat was studied in blue light, red light with fluorescent dyes.

She studied the electrical behavior of the unsaturated fatty acids and their "halo" using rhodamine red dyes. With this technique she proved that electron rich highly unsaturated Linoleic and Linolenic fatty acids were the undiscovered mysterious decisive fats in respiratory enzyme function that Otto Warburg had been unable to find. She studied the electromagnetic function of pi-electrons of the linolenic acid in the membranes of the microstructure of protoplasm, for all nerve

78

function, secretions, mitosis, as well as cell break-down. This immediately caused lot of excitement in the scientific community. New doors could open in Cancer research. Hydrogenated fats, including all trans fatty acids were proved to be respiratory poisons.

Dr. Budwig found that the blood of seriously ill cancer patients was deficient in these unsaturated omega-3 fats, lipoproteins, phosphatides, and hemoglobin. In addition, she also noticed that cancer patients had a strange greenish-yellow substance in their blood that she could not find in the blood of healthy people. Budwig proposed a treatment program for cancer based on two simple ingredients: flaxseed oil and cottage cheese.

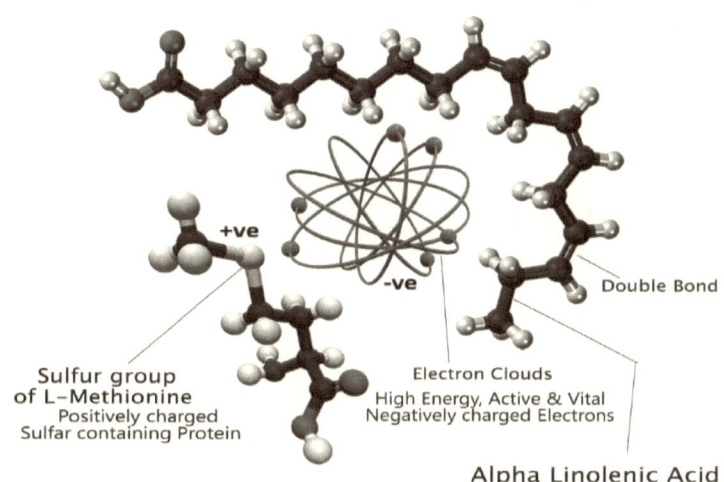

Bonding of Alpha-Linolenic Acid ALA and Sulfurated Protein

+ve

-ve

Double Bond

Sulfur group
of L-Methionine
Positively charged
Sulfar containing Protein

Electron Clouds
High Energy, Active & Vital
Negatively charged Electrons

Alpha Linolenic Acid

Then Budwig decided to have human trials and selected the cancer patients from four Hospitals in Münster. She gave flaxseed oil and quark to these patients. After three months, the patients began to improve in health and strength, the yellow green substance in their blood began to disappear, tumors gradually receded and at the same time the nutrients began to rise. This way Dr. Budwig had found a cure for cancer. It was a great victory and first milestone in the battle against cancer. Her treatment protocol is based on the consumption of flaxseed oil with low fat cottage cheese, raw organic diet, mild exercise, and the healing powers of the sun. She treated approx. 2500 cancer patients during a 50 year period with this protocol till her death with over 90% documented success, even in the terminal and hopeless cancer patients rejected by allopathy (Budwig, Cancer The Problem And The Solution).

She was nominated 7 times for Nobel Prize but with a condition that she will use chemotherapy and radiotherapy with her protocol. They did not want to collapse the 200 billion business over night. She always refused to support the damaging chemo and radio for the sake of humanity.

Dr. Johanna Budwig's Works in English

- FlaxOil As A True Aid Against Arthritis, Heart Infarction, Cancer, And Other Diseases by Dr. Johanna Budwig
- The Oil-Protein Diet Cookbook The Oil-Protein Diet Cookbook by Dr. Johanna Budwig
- Dr Budwig: Cancer - The Problem and The Solution by Dr Johanna Budwig

Federal Institute where Dr. Budwig worked

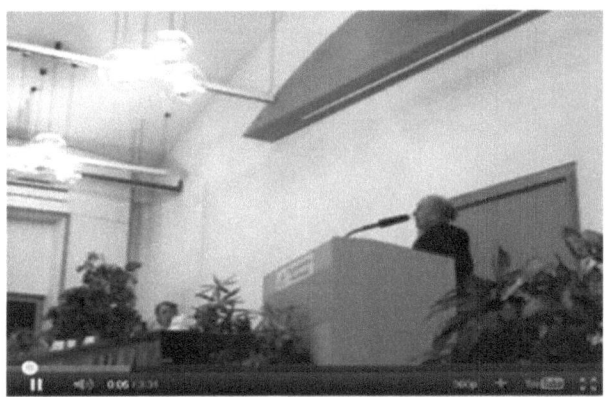

This is a rare picture of Dr. Budwig during her last public lecture in Freudenstadt, Germany. This lecture was a Birth day gift to Mr. Lothar Hirneise.

There are many organizations to get involved with for everyone who believes in this. And those who want to join the effort should strive to do it.

She reiterates the importance of the work they are doing. She is convinced that the efforts made by the pioneers are being continued in such places as Australia, where doctors of medicine, chemistry and teachers carry on the work. They have asked her to come and teach them, but she said that at 90 years old that is not what she wants to do at this point. (...)

Over fifty years ago, Johanna Budwig was the first to highlight the benefits of "omega-3 " and the evils of transfat, which are being " rediscovered " today. But her name remains virtually unknown to scientists, the media and the general public.

These are pictures are of the **"Bundesanstalt Fur Fettforschung"**, the **Federal Institute for Fat Research** in Germany where Dr. Budwig worked at. It explains that the Institute contributed largely to the connection between saturated and unsaturated fats. The video says that the woman who made the decisive discovery was Dr. Budwig, who showed the difference between the saturated and unsaturated fats. She was

81

against the margarine industry and said that it caused cancer and other diseases.

She made many discoveries at the Institute of Fats Research and while working with Professor Kaufman (Escher).

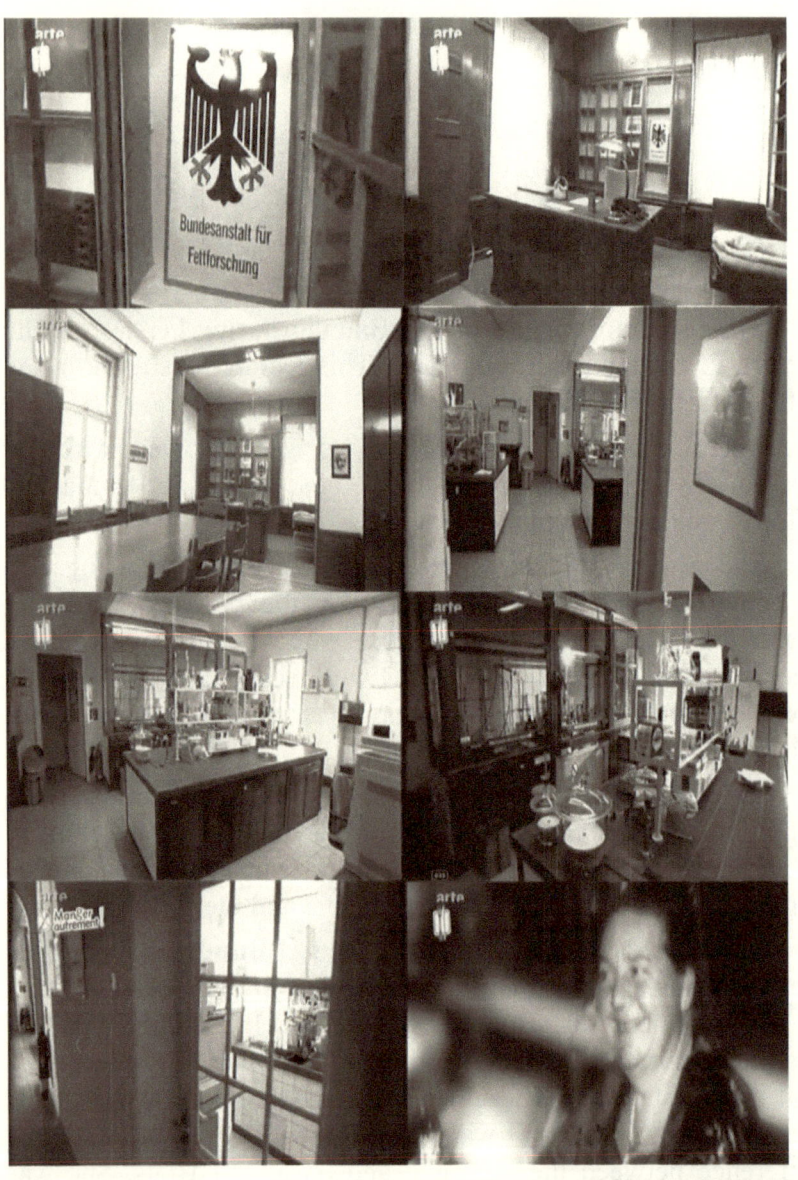

Budwig Protocol

Transition Diet

The Transition diet is especially recommended for patients of liver, pancreatic or gall bladder cancers. The basic principle is that for 3 days nothing is eaten and drunk except the following written and at least three times daily warm tea (herbal teas from peppermint, rose hip, mallow or green tea) is drunk. Dr Budwig has recommended variant 1 for patients with a relatively good energy state, and variant 2 and 3 mainly for seriously ill patients.

Variant 1

Variant 1 for three days, 250 g of linomel or alternatively freshly crushed Flax seed is eaten together with the following:

- Freshly pressed fruit juices without added sugar.
- Freshly pressed vegetable juices such as carrot, celery juice, red beetroots and apple juice.
- Chinese tea and black tea are allowed in the morning
- Honey for sweetening is allowed. Just as grape juice for drinking and as a sweetener. Energetically weak patients can also consume sparkling wine and linomel.

Variant 2

For three days, oat meal cereal very hour with linomel is eaten daily with the following juices:

- Freshly pressed fruit juices or freshly pressed vegetable juices such as carrot, celery juice, beetroot and apple juice.
- Chinese tea and black tea are allowed in the morning.
- Honey for sweetening is allowed. Just as grape juice for drinking and as a sweetener.
- Energetically weak patients can also consume sparkling wine and linomel.

Variant 3

For three days, oatmeal soup with linomel is given three times a day together with the following juices:

- Freshly pressed fruit juices or fruit juices without added sugar.
- Freshly pressed vegetable juices such as carrot, celery juice, beetroot and apple juice.
- Chinese tea and black tea are allowed in the morning.
- Honey for sweetening is allowed. Just as grape juice for drinking and as a sweetener.
- Energetically weak patients can also consume sparkling wine and linomel.

It is often experienced frequently that patients mixed all three variants and "nevertheless" had good results. So better you to stick to one variant. (Budwig – Cancer The Problem And The Solution 2005: p.36).

Budwig Diet

The Budwig Protocol is one of the most widely followed alternative treatments for cancer and other diseases. The diet seems simple, but foods are powerful and can heal a person.

6:00 AM – Sauerkraut juice

A glass of sauerkraut juice consumed before breakfast every morning. It is rich in vitamins including C, enzymes and helps develop the health-promoting gut flora. Sauerkraut is cabbage that has been pickled by natural fermentation, mainly with lactobacillus bacteria. It is slightly salty, sharp and sour. Well made, it is much nicer than it sounds. You may also consume another glass of sauerkraut juice later in the day.

It interesting that sauerkraut contains right rotating lactic acids and is highly alkaline and neutralizes levo-rotating lactic acids and makes our body alkaline. That is why Marcus Porcius Cato the Elder issued a statement - Carcinomas are incurable except with the treatment with Sauerkraut.

8:00 AM Breakfast

Herbal tea

Start breakfast with a cup of warm herbal or green tea. Sweeten with only natural honey. You can add lemon or grape juice. Patient should take such a tea half an hour before each meal. He may consume 4-5 teas in a day.

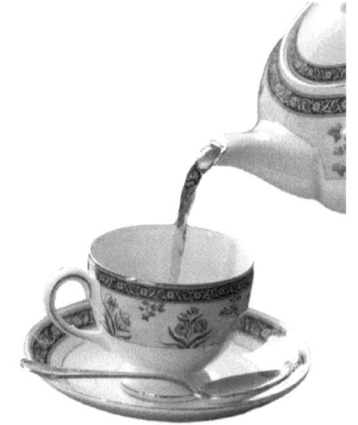

Linomel Muesli or Oil-Protein Muesli

This should be made fresh and consumed within 15 minutes. It is full of high energy pi-electrons, attract oxygen in the cells and capable of healing cell membranes. It is full of energy-rich omega-3 fats, has power to attract healing photons from sun through resonance. As "Om" is divine word and synonym of God in India. According to Hindu Mythology, the whole universe is located inside "Om", so the name Omkhand has been given to this wonderful recipe in Hindi.

Ingredients

- 3 Tbsp cold pressed organic Flax seed oil (FO)
- 100-125gm (6 Tbsp) Quark or Cottage Cheese(CC)
- 2 Tbsp freshly ground Flax seeds
- 2 Tbsp milk
- 1 cup fruits
- ¼ cup dried nuts
- Natural honey
- Flavorings – lemon, apple cider vinegar, cinnamon, pure cacao, natural vanilla, shredded coconut etc.

Recipe

Place 2 tablespoons Linomel or freshly ground Flax seeds in a small bowl. It is covered with raw, crushed or diced seasonal fruits depending on the season. Pour some orange or grape juice over this. Linomel^{Tm} is a brand name 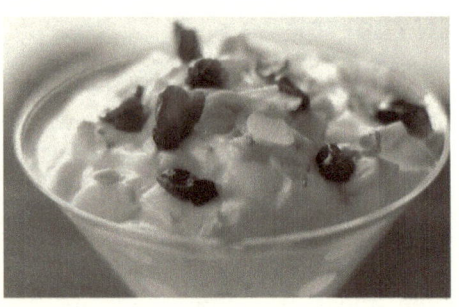 and originally created and patented by Budwig. It is a cereal made from cracked Flax Seed, a small amount of honey and a little milk powder.

Then the Quark-Flax seed oil cream is prepared in as follows: First add Flax seed oil, milk and honey and blend briefly with a hand-held immersion electric blender, then gradually add the Quark in smaller portions. Blend till oil and Quark is thoroughly mixed with no separated oil. Then it is seasoned differently everyday with different flavorings such as vanilla, cinnamon or various fruits such as banana, apple, lemon, orange juice, or berries.

Use various fruits such as fresh berries, apple, cherry, orange, banana, papaya, grapes etc. Add other fresh fruit if you like, totaling 1/2 to 1 cup of fruit. Budwig specially advised to use berries like strawberry, blueberry, raspberry, cheery 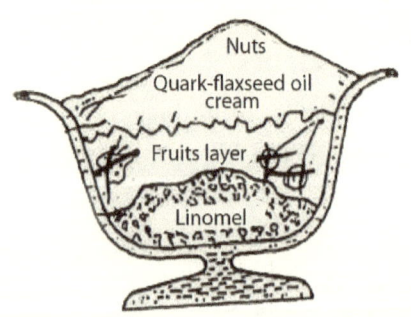 etc. because berries have ellagic acids which are strong cancer fighters.

Add organic raw nuts such as walnuts, almonds, raisins or Brazil nuts. They have sulfurated proteins, omega-3 fats and vitamins. Brazil nut is especially important because a single nut provides you with all of the selenium you need for the day. Selenium is very important to boost immune power. Peanuts are prohibited.

For variety and flavor, try natural vanilla, cinnamon, lemon juice, pure cocoa or shredded coconut.

Once blended in Budwig Cream, Quark and Flax seed oil form a new substance called lipoprotein. Lipoprotein is a water soluble complex. The Quark is rich in the sulfur-containing amino acids, methionine and cysteine. These positively charged amino acids attract the negatively charged electron clouds in fatty acid chains and exhibit a stabilizing effect on the highly unsaturated, otherwise easily oxidized fats. Thus, the amino acids protect the polyunsaturated fatty acids from the Flax seed oil against oxidation which, as a result, are able to enter the human body unchanged and with their full energy potential. The result: they are much more valuable to cells and their membranes. Consequently, one could say that Quark excels as a protector for the polyunsaturated fatty acids.

Sulfur-rich amino acids play a wealth of roles in many vital functions in our bodies. In combination with polyunsaturated fatty acids, they are important partners in regulating the uptake of oxygen and its utilization by the cell. They therefore contribute significantly to a strong immune system, healthy metabolism, and mental vitality. For many generations, people have been getting their omega-3 fatty acids from fish, vegetables, nuts, and seeds. Our health literally depends on the regular consumption of the essential

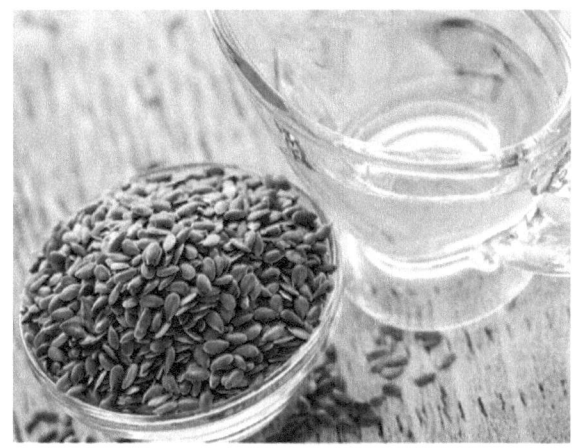

omega-3 and omega-6 fatty acids, alpha-linolenic acid (ALA) and linoleic acid (LA). Our bodies require these fatty acids in order to synthesize their cell membranes as well as for a variety of metabolic processes and heal the cancer and other diseases.

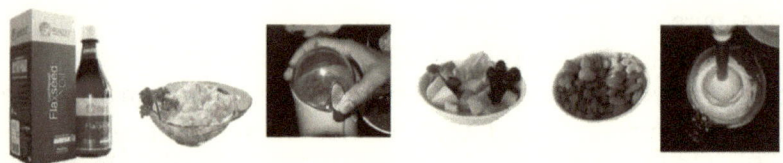

Tips for making the Budwig Mixture

- Follow directions properly! It is important to add things to the mixture in the right order. If you mix them in the wrong order you may lose a lot of the opportunity to convert the oil-soluble omega-3 into water soluble-omega-3.
- Keep the Flax seed oil refrigerated.
- Immersion blender is a must.
- The mixture can be flavored differently every day by adding nuts and fruits preferably organic such as pecans, almonds or walnuts (not peanuts), banana, organic cocoa, shredded coconut, pineapple (fresh) blueberries, raspberries, cinnamon, vanilla or (freshly) squeezed fruit juice.
- Consume immediately for best results.

10 AM Vegetable juice

Freshly squeezed vegetable juice from carrots, beets, celery, tomato, and radish, lemon as well as green vegetables - stinging nettle, lettuce or spinach. Apple is added to sweeten and enhance the taste. Carrot & beet juices are especially helpful to the liver and have strong cancer fighting properties. Vary vegetables. Some tasty and nutritious combinations are beet and apple juice, carrot and apple, carrot and beet, asparagus and apple, celery and apple, celery and carrot. Beet juice should not be taken alone. If taken alone it may cause red or pink urine (beeturia).

She also frequently recommended the following juices:

1. Nettle juice - Especially in the spring, Dr Budwig recommended to puree nettles with water and a lemon.

2. Radish juice - For this, a radish is first crushed and then thrown together with a lemon into the juicer. This juice is by the way durable for several days and Dr Budwig has sometimes recommended her patients to drink a small quantity of them every day.

3. Coltsfoot juice - For this juice, with the exception of the harder old rootstock, the entire remaining underground shoot is mixed with a few flowers and some milk and honey.

4. Horseradish juice - Mix 3-5 cm horseradish together with an apple and (raw) milk. Depending on the quantity of milk you can change the taste. Dr Budwig recommended this juice above all to workmen and to stimulate the appetite. Freshly pressed means, by the way, that you drink the juice within 5 minutes after pressing. In some cases, Dr Budwig prescribed a second juice 30 to 60 minutes later.

10 AM Vegetable juice

Freshly squeezed vegetable juice from carrots, beets, celery, tomato, and radish, lemon as well as green vegetables - stinging nettle, lettuce or spinach. Apple is added to sweeten and enhance the taste. Carrot & beet juices are especially helpful to the liver and have strong cancer fighting properties. Vary vegetables. Some tasty and nutritious combinations are beet and apple juice, carrot and apple, carrot and beet, asparagus and apple, celery and apple, celery and carrot. Beet juice should not be taken alone. If taken alone it may cause red or pink urine (beeturia).

12:15 PM Lunch

Salad Platter: Salad plate with homemade cottage cheese-flaxseed mayonnaise. As salad also use: dandelion, cress, celery, tomato, cucumber, lettuce, radish, cabbage, broccoli, green horseradish and pepper.

Delicious mayo salad dressing can be prepared by mixing together 2 Tbsp (30 ml) Flax Oil, 2 Tbsp (30 ml) milk, and 2 Tbsp (30 ml) cottage cheese. Then add 2 tablespoons (30 ml) of Lemon juice (or Apple Cider Vinegar) and add 1 teaspoon 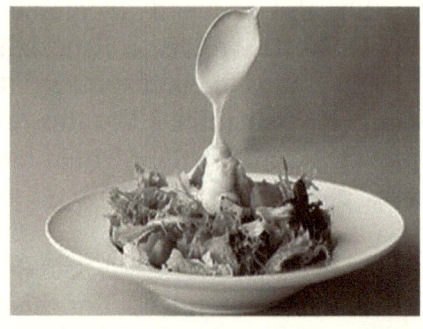 (2.5g) Mustard powder plus some herbs of your choice. Other alternative dressing can be made by mixing Flax Oil, lemon juice, Mustard and some herbs (Budwig, The Oil-Protein Diet Cookbook, 1994).

Main Course: Vegetables cooked in water, then flavored with Oleolox and herbs possibly with oatmeal, soy sauce, curry etc. Vegetable broth flavored with a little Oleolox and yeast flakes. As side dish for the vegetables: buckwheat, brown rice, millet or potatoes can be used. One or two slices of Ezekiel bread can be taken. Use lot of dried fruits in the main meal also.

Lunch Dessert: Cottage cheese/ Flax oil mixture served as a sweet dish prepared with dry fruits and fruits such as pineapple, or poured over a fruit salad. You already know how to prepare it perfectly.

3 PM Fruit juice

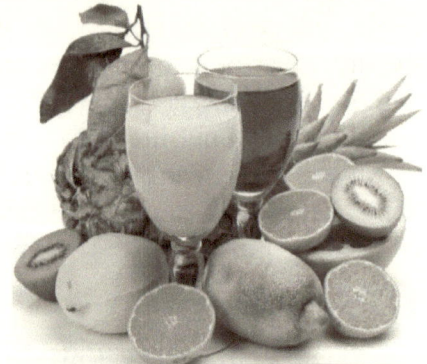

Consume 1 glass grape, cherry, pomegranate juice, orange juice or organic Champagne with 2 tablespoon freshly ground flaxseed.

3:30 PM Enzyme Fruit juice

Consume pure pineapple or papaya juice with 2 tablespoon freshly ground flaxseed.

6 PM Dinner

The evening meal should be light and served early, around 6 p.m. A warm meal may be prepared using brown rice, buckwheat or oat meal. Never consume corn or soy beans. Dishes made with buckwheat grouts are most easily tolerated and nourishing. Use only honey 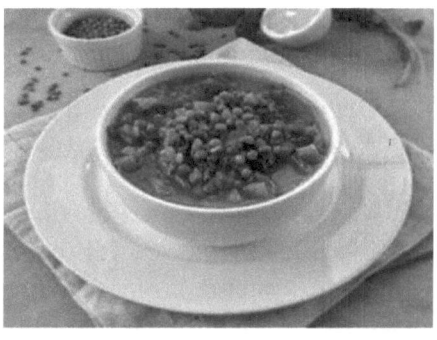 to sweeten. Soup or more solid dishes can be combined with a tasty sauce according to preference. Use OLEOLOX liberally also to sweet sauces and soups, making them nourishing and a richer source of energy.

8:30 PM

A glass of organic red wine or champagne may be consumed. All things are a matter of correct dosage. In fact, seriously ill patients having pain and discomfort just starting on the oil-protein diet, it is recommended to serve a glass of champagne mixed with freshly ground flaxseeds to tide them over while going off pain killers (Budwig, Cancer The Problem And The Solution).

Precautions

Reverse Osmosis (R.O.) filtered water- Use RO water for drinking, cooking and enemas.

Eat Organic Diet - Always try to eat organic food.

Dental Care –

Mercury is a Carcinogenic as well as a Poison! The root canals of dead teeth are full of bacteria that attack the liver and lymphatic system. From Amalgam fillings the mercury slowly leaks out of the filings. The ADA cleverly defends the use of amalgam in spite of the fact that there is sufficient evidence that patients with many severe problems, including psychotic episodes and fatal allergic reactions, were just cured by removing the amalgam. It is advisable to rather have a ceramic filling than be slowly poisoned by mercury. Even gold filling is dangerous; it acts as battery producing electrical current. Be informed that the effect of drugs, including poison, is dose dependant and cumulative.

Fluoride is not only toxic but it is also carcinogenic. Fluoride has never been proven to prevent tooth decay. It has been outlawed in many countries or groups of countries because the evidence is overwhelming that fluoride causes premature aging, so drink bottled water and use fluoride-free toothpaste (American Cancer Institute - 1963).

I highly recommend helping you avoid fillings in the first place. Holistic dentist recommend 3% H_2O_2 as a gargle or rinse, or making a paste using baking soda. H_2O_2 usage three times a day is advised. It is great for cleaning dentures, too.

Frying and deep frying

Frying and deep frying is not allowed to cook patient's food. Never heat any oil in the kitchen. By heating oils the wealth of high energy electrons is destroyed and trans fats and dangerous toxic chemicals such as acrylamides are formed in the oil. Boiling and steaming are good practices. You can fry vegetables etc. in water and add oleolox before serving. Water is the safest medium for frying, says Lothar Hirneise.

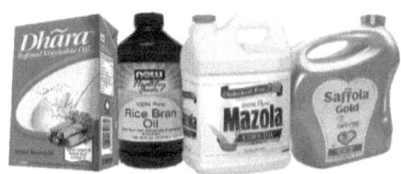

Chemo and Radio

Chemotherapy is aimed at destruction of the tumor, and it destroys many living cells, and the entire person. Anything that disturbs growth is fatal because growth is an elementary function of life. We cannot achieve something good with bad tools.

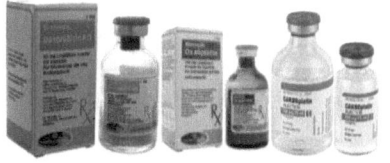

Dr. Budwig rejects Chemo and Radiation Therapy. Budwig used to say with full confidence and clarity, "My treatment attacks on the real cause of cancer; it fills cancer cells with high energy pi-electrons and attracts oxygen into the cells. And cancer cells start to breathe and produce vital energy. Thus cancer suffocates in presence of oxygen and start to die."

Man-made Supplements

With this treatment man-made antioxidants, synthetic vitamins and pain killers should not be given. The dose of anticoagulants and aspirin should be adjusted by your doctor. Dr. Budwig favors natural, herbal and homeopathy instead of man-made and synthetic supplements, vitamins and pain killers (Budwig, Cancer The Problem And The Solution).

Prohibitions of Budwig Protocol

In this protocol there are certain restrictions. They are as important as the diet itself. It is very difficult to defeat the cancer without strictly following these rules.

Sugar is strictly forbidden

Jiggery, molasses, maple syrup and artificial sweeteners like xylitol, aspartame are not permitted. You can use only unprocessed natural honey, stevia and fruit juices.

Be Vegetarian

Meat, fish, poultry, eggs, butter and ghee are never allowed. Preserved meat is like a poison. It is highly processed and treated with dangerous antibiotics, preservatives and nitrates.

Stop using Hydrogenated Fat and Refined oil

You can never eat pizza, burger, fast food, fried food, biscuits, samosa etc. as they all are made by hydrogenated margarine and shortenings. Hydrogenation is a very dangerous process, used to increase shelf life of fats. In this process (in which oil is heated at very high temperature and Hydrogen is passed through oils in presence of nickel) killing trans fats are formed, high energy live and vital electrons are destroyed and nutrients are damaged. Hydrogenated Fat is just a dead, nutrition less and cancer causing liquid plastic. Budwig always preached against these damaging fats. She has allowed low fat cheese, oleolox and coconut oil.

Preservatives and Processed Food

You should not eat Potato chips, soft drinks etc. which are full of preservatives. Never consume highly processed food like ready to eat packed foods, pasta, pastries, bread and soy products, tofu etc. But good quality soy souse is permitted.

Microwave, Teflon, Aluminum and Plastic

Never cook in microwave oven. Food cooked in microwave become toxic and deformed. Also don't use aluminum, plastic,

Teflon coated cookware and aluminum foils. Use stainless steel, iron, china clay or glass utensils instead.

Chemicals and pesticides are not allowed

Avoid pesticides and chemicals, even those in household products & cosmetics. Stay away from mosquito repellants, sun screen lotions and sun glasses.

Wear natural fibers

Don't wear clothes made using synthetic fiber like nylon, polyester and acrylic. Wear cotton, wool or silk instead. Don't use on foam pillow and mattress.

CRT TV and mobile phones

These emit dangerous electromagnetic radiation, so do not use them. You can watch LCD and plasma TVs.

No left over

Food should be prepared fresh and eaten soon after preparation to maximize intake of health giving electrons and enzymes (Budwig, Cancer The Problem And The Solution).

Eldi oil

Dr. Budwig created unique Eldi oils, called Electron Differential Oils after performing precise spectroscopic measurements of the light absorption in different oils - specifying that the oils contained pi-electron clouds from flax oil, wheat germ oil plus vitamin-E in its natural complex, etheric oils and sulfhydryl groups.

Dr. Johanna Budwig said, "The sun is my preferred treatment modality, as is Eldi oil, used externally to stimulate the absorption of the long-wave band of the sun. I have used ELDI oils extensively since 1968 for 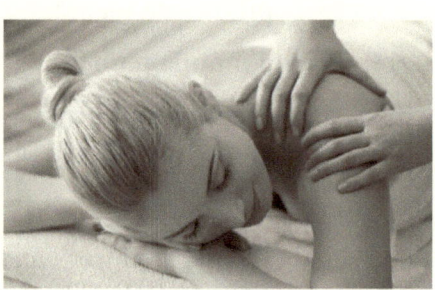 body massage as well as in the selective application of oil packs. US pain institute has written somewhere: 'What this crazy woman does with her ELDI oils, none of us manages to do via pain killers." Dr. Budwig has clearly mentioned that if Eldi oil is not available you may use flax oil instead.

Massage Benefits

- Since ancient time massage has been part of cancer healing. Think of your lymphatics as a trash-disposal system for your body. Massage initiates lymphatic drainage, you push the trash out of your body and you're helping your immune system.
- Massage therapy is sometimes the first really pleasant touch a patient is able to experience.
- Massage also releases endorphins (our body's natural painkillers), stimulates lymph movement, and stretches tissues throughout the body. It's energizing, stimulating, and pretty good feeling.

Procedure –

Two times a day, i.e. morning and evening, rub Eldi Oil R or flax oil into the skin over the whole body, a bit more intensely on the shoulders, armpits and groin area (where plenty lymphatic vessels are present) as well as the problem areas, such as the breast, stomach, liver, etc. Leave the oil on the skin for about 20 minutes and follow with a warm shower without washing with soap. After 10 minutes take another shower, this time using a mild soap, and then rest for 15-20 minutes.

The purpose of the shower

Once the body has been oiled and the Eldi Oil or flax oil has penetrated the skin, the warm water will open the pores and the oil may penetrate the skin more deeply. The second shower, where one washes with soap, cleanses the skin so that clothes and linen will not become overly soiled.

Oil Packs

Take a piece of cloth made of pure cotton. Cut to a size to fit the body part, such as the knee. Soak the cotton cloth with oil, place on the knee etc., cover it with a plastic sheet and wrap it up with an elastic bandage. Leave overnight. Remove in the morning and wash the knee; repeat in the evening. Keep applying the same procedure for weeks, you get good results. You can use Eldi Oil R, flax oil or castor oil for these local applications. The oil pack is only suitable for local problems (no metastases).

Oil Enema

Dr Budwig used to give eldi oil R or flax oil enema to her serious patients. Dr. Budwig used to get immediate and miraculous results with the most seriously ill patients. ELDI oil and Flaxseed Oil give very similar results.

Ingredients

- Enema pot
- Watch

- A bowl to collect oil when you are getting rid of bubbles.
- Towel and tissue
- RO filtered water
- Eldi oil or flax oil
- Towel or Drip Stand

Procedure

Prepare a spot near the toilet, so that if you can't hold the enema you will be making a quick dash and the shorter distance is better.

Cleansing Enema with Plain water

First of all you should take a plain water enema. Purpose of this enema is cleansing of intestines. It is not a retention enema and is evacuated immediately. For this you may use 500-1000 ml (2-4 cups) RO filtered water. As soon as the whole water is inside the rectum, go and sit on the commode and release the water slowly.

Take the oil enema immediately after the water enema

- Use 200-250 ml of eldi or flax oil. The oil should be at body temperature. The best test is to dip your little finger into the oil.
- Fill the oil into the enema pot. It takes at least 5 minutes for the bubbles to get out of the tube.
- The enema pot should be hanged on a drip stand about 2-3 feet above your body.
- You need to lubricate the nozzle and anus with flax oil. When all is ready, lie on your right side in the fetal position. Insert the nozzle into the rectum slowly and carefully with your left hand, and un-pinch the tube.
- If you feel little uncomfortable when the oil is going in, pinch the tube, wait till the feeling passes away, then continue again.

- The oil is much more viscous and moves more slowly. You might need to hold the pot a bit higher to get it to run a bit quicker.
- Once the oil is in, wait and hold it for about 12-15 minutes. After that slowly turn yourself to left side and hold oil for another 12-15 minutes. You may listen to music while taking enema.
- When done, it is best to sit on the commode for about 15 minutes with something to read (Skelton).

Coffee Enema

Dr. Max Gerson introduced coffee enema back in the 1930s. In this enema 2 to 3 cups of coffee is pushed into rectum, but coffee only reaches up to sigmoid colon. There is no loss of 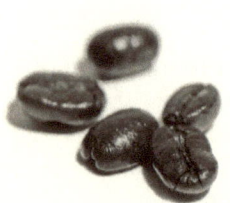 minerals and electrolytes in Coffee Enema because their absorption occurs well before sigmoid colon. Coffee enema is even safe for those who are allergic to coffee because it is not absorbed into the systemic circulation. It has the following benefits.

- **Powerful and Natural Pain Reliever**
- **Cleansing** - Coffee also acts as an astringent in the large intestine, helping clean the colon walls.
- **Toxin Elimination** - The major benefit of the coffee enema is elimination of toxins through the liver. Caffeine, theophylline and theobromine dilate blood vessels and bile ducts, stimulate the liver to discharge bile and boost the detoxifying process into high gear and heal inflammation. Indeed, endoscopic studies confirm they increase bile output.
- **Stimulates Liver** - Kahweol and cafestol palmitate found in coffee promote the activity of a key enzyme system called glutathione S-transferase. This is an important mechanism in the detoxification of carcinogens, as the enzyme group is responsible for neutralizing free radicals. Coffee enema stimulates the activity of this system by 600- 700%.

Coffee Enema Procedure

- This enema is retained for 12-15 minutes, during this time blood circulates in liver three times and blood is purified. Coffee enema can be given several times a day, few patients take up to seven times a day. Normally if pain is not relieved he may take more than one time. You should relax while taking enema; you may listen to music or read newspaper while relaxing. The best time for coffee enema is either early morning after you passed motion or during the day time.

- Grind 2-3 Tbsp organic coffee beans. It is roughly 25 grams. Put 800-1000 ml of filtered water in a steal pan and bring it to boil. Add 2-5 Tbsp coffee powder. Let it continue to simmer for ten minutes or more and then turn off the burner. Allow it to cool down to a very comfortable, tepid temperature. Test it with your finger. It should be the same temperature as your body's temperature. Filter the coffee with fine mesh steal sieve into a jug.

- Pour 2 cups of coffee into the enema pot. Be sure the plastic hose is clamped tightly. Now open the clamp and grasp, but do not close the clamp on the hose. Place the enema tip in the sink. Hold up the enema bag above the tip until the coffee begins to flow out. As soon as it starts flowing, quickly close the clamp. This expels any air in the tube.

- Lubricate the enema tip with a small amount of coconut oil. Create a comfortable and relaxing atmosphere. After a few days you will thoroughly enjoy this ritual.

- Light a candle, play some light music and most importantly, make sure you are comfortable and warm. We recommend placing a pillow with a washable cover under your head and lying down on a large, dark towel.

- The position preferred is lying on your back on the floor. With the clamp closed hang the pot about 3 feet above your belly. We like to hang the enema pot on a drip stand.

- Insert the tip gently into anus and open the clamp slowly. You should relax and breathe. The coffee may take a few seconds to begin flowing. If you develop a cramp, close the hose clamp, turn from side to side and take a few deep breaths. The cramp will usually pass quickly.

- When all the liquid is inside, close the clamp and remove it slowly. Retain the enema for 12- 14 minutes. You may remain lying on the floor.

- After 14 minutes or so, go to the toilet and empty your gut. Take your time. Wash the enema pot and tube thoroughly with soap and water.

- Take more potassium in the form of fruits and vegetable juices if you take coffee enema regularly (S.A.Wilsons.com).

Epsom bath

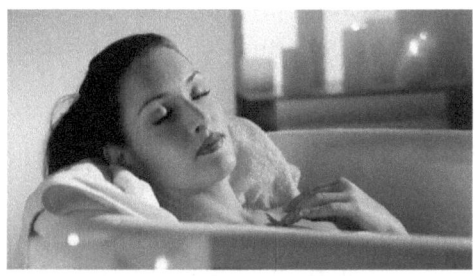

Detoxification of your body through bathing is an ancient remedy that anyone can perform in the comfort of your own home. Your skin is known as the third kidney, and toxins are excreted through sweating. An Epsom bath is thought to assist your body in eliminating toxins as well as absorbing the magnesium and nutrients that are in the water. Soaking in Epsom salt actually helps replenish the body's magnesium levels, combating hypertension. The sulfate flushes toxins and helps form proteins in brain tissue and joints. Most of all, it will leave you relaxed, refreshed and awakened. Take it once a week.

Prepare your bath

It is a 40 minutes ritual. The first 20 minutes are said to help your body remove the toxins, while the second 20 minutes are for absorbing the minerals from the water

- Fill your tub with comfortably hot water. Use a chlorine filter if possible.
- Add Epsom salt (Magnesium sulfate). For people 50 Kg and up, add 2 cups or more to a standard bath tub.
- Then add 1 to 2 cups or more of soda bicarb. It is known for its cleansing ability and even has anti-fungal properties. It also leaves skin very soft.
- Add ground ginger. While this step is optional, ginger can increase your heat levels, helping to sweat out more toxins. However, since it is heating the body, it may cause your skin to turn slightly red for a few minutes, so be careful with the amount you add. Depending on the

capacity of your tub, anywhere from 1 Tbsp to 1/3 cup can be added (Herneise).

- Add aromatherapy oils. Again optional, but there are many oils that will make the bath an even more pleasant and relaxing experience (such as lavender), as well as those that will assist in the detoxification process (tea tree oil or eucalyptus oil). Around 20 drops is sufficient for a standard bath.

- Swish all of the ingredients around in the tub, and then slip into the tub. You should start sweating within the first few minutes. If you feel too hot, start adding cold water into the tub until you cool off.

- Get out of the tub slowly and carefully. Your body has been working hard and you may get lightheaded or feel weak and drained. On top of that, the salts make your tub slippery, so stand with care.

- Drink plenty of water and relax in bed for a few minutes

Soda bicarb bath

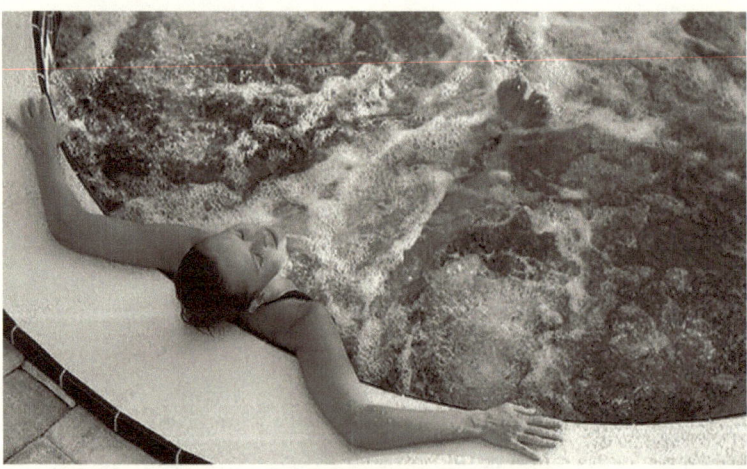

Lothar Hirneise has given lot of importance to Soda bicarb bath. It is thought to assist you in eliminating toxins as well as making your body alkaline so your tumor cells suffocate. Patient may take it once or even twice a day. Just add 2 cups of soda bicarb in your bath tub filled with warm water and relax in it for 30-40 minutes (Hirneise, 2005).

Sun Therapy

Getting an adequate amount of sunshine is a critical part of Budwig protocol. Once the body has acquired the right oil-protein balance with the cottage cheese and flax oil, the body develops better absorption to access the healing powers of the sun. The sunshine is important to maintain adequate vitamin-D levels in our body. Vitamin-D is a powerful antioxidant that has been linked to preventing many diseases including cancer.

Dr. Budwig's focus was on the importance of photons from the sunbeams and their interaction with vital essential fats (linoleic and linolenic acid) in our body. It is the interaction of photons from the sun and the electrons in proper food that provide the synergistic effect on healing our body. Eating the electron rich flax oil/cottage cheese mixture, must be connected with adequate exposure to sunlight.

There is nothing else on earth with a higher concentration of photons of the sun's energy than man. This concentration of the sun's energy is very much energetic point for humans, with their eminently suitable wave lengths - is improved when we eat electron rich essential oils which in turn attract the electro-magnetic waves of sun beams, the photons.

When you eat the FO/CC mixture, your body becomes a better antenna for the photons from the sun. Your body develops a better ability to absorb the energy from the sun and transfer it to your cells to perform their vital functions. You become energized at a deep level, and when this happens cancer is healed itself.

Oleolox – Budwig butter

Oleolox (Oleolox – Oleo = oil & Lux = Light) is full of sun photons. It is best and tasty substitute of Butter proposed by Budwig.

105

Recipe -

- Pour cool 125 ml flaxseed oil in a wide mouth bottle and keep it in the refrigerator.

- In a stainless steel pan, heat 250 g coconut oil.

- Add a medium sized onion (roughly 100 grams) cut in 2 pieces. Cook about 7-10 minutes until the onion is slightly browned.

- Then add 10 garlic cloves.

- Heat the garlic for about 3 minutes in the pan with the onion.

- When the onion and garlic are fried in the coconut oil; the protective qualities of the sulfur present in the onion and garlic are transferred to coconut oil. This in turn protects the flaxseed oil. Remove the onion and garlic. Leave the coconut oil to cool down.

- Pour the coconut oil through a sieve into the cooled FO.

- Keep the Oleolox in the refrigerator.

Use it as a spread on Ezekiel bread or chapatti, potatoes and other vegetables. For the best results, the boil or steam vegetables, after being cooked, should be coated with Oleolox. In Oil-Protein cook book Budwig advises that Oleolox should never be heated more than one or two minutes. Use a clock/timer to make sure you don't overheat the Oleolox (Budwig, The Oil-Protein Diet Cookbook, 1994).

Rebounder

Your body has about 60 trillion cells. The gravitational pull involved in bouncing on a "Rebounder" squeezes out toxins. Then, during the brief weightless period when the body is suspended in the air, the lower pressure in the

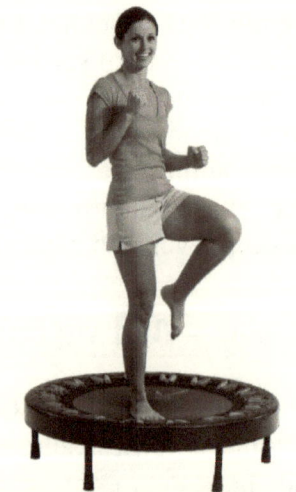

cell promotes the movement of nutrients into the cells. Thus the flow of materials to and from cells is improved. It is like getting every cell in your body to exercise.

Mild exercise

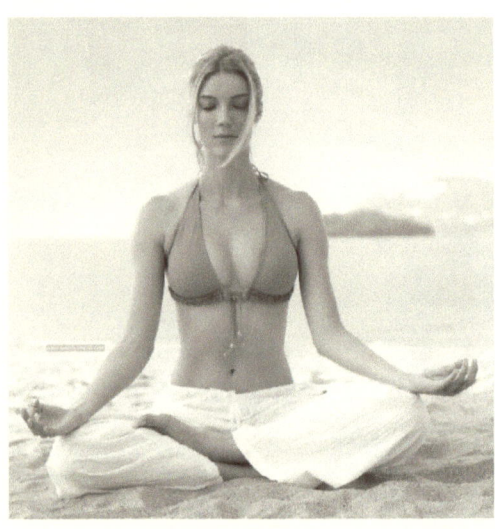

Patient can do mild exercise and remain active if his condition permits. He can go for a walk or do light yoga in the open terrace or garden under the healing and refreshing sunshine. Patient can jog for a few minutes after lunch or dinner. It is very beneficial for cancer patient. But if patient is serious and has metastasis, he should not jog, better he should relax in his house.

Patient can keep himself busy in many activities like sitting in garden enjoying nature, visualization, listening music, reading, laughing, chatting with friends etc. Stress, depression, anxiety, anger and fear can be very damaging to him. Share your feelings with your life partner or a best friend.

You should try your best to remove stress and negative thoughts and balance the flow of energy "chi" in your body. Do meditation, Emotional Freedom Technique EFT, Qigong, Reiki, Acupuncture, Acupressure, Sun Salutation etc. to heal your body, mind and spirit.

Meditation

Meditation is a means of transforming the mind. Meditation practices are techniques that encourage and develop concentration, clarity, positivity, and relaxation of the body and mind. Do any simple Meditation for relaxation.

Yoga Nidra

It is divine sleep with alertness. In 20 minute Yoga Nidra session, you relax in a fully supported corpse pose (Shavasana pose), limbs limp, breath quiet, thoughts drifting by. In the distance, the teacher's voice blends with the sound of Tibetan bells. All 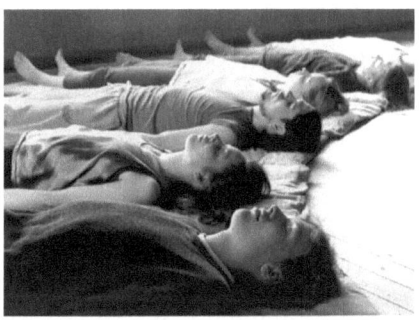 traces of the day fade away, time stops, and stillness washes over the body. Yoga Nidra is a systematic method of complete relaxation, holistically addressing our physiological, neurological, and subconscious needs.

Juicing for the Budwig Protocol

"Juicing", making your own fresh juices, is one of the important cornerstones of the Budwig Protocol. There is no point in overloading on one fruit or vegetable juice; so try to get plenty of variety in the juices you drink.

Juices specifically recommended by Dr Johanna Budwig include carrot, celery and apple, beet and apple, radish, cherry grape, pomegranate and red currant and stinging nettle.

Mix and combine your juices to taste. Juices are best made with good, fresh and preferably organic fruit and vegetables. They should be drunk as fresh as possible to ensure the vitamins and enzymes are still active. It is always best to press it yourself for that meal.

Nettle juice is rich in vitamin C and always been a folk remedy for cleansing the blood.

Almost all fruit and vegetables, leaves such as spinach, chard or watercress or even wheat and barley grass can be pressed.

Budwig Diet Juicing Routine

Early morning you must have a glass of sauerkraut juice.

Breakfast: Juice can be used to moisten ground linseed or add flavor to the quark-linseed oil cream for breakfast in muesli or add a cup of juice to the ground linseed, quark-linseed oil cream, liquidize the fresh fruits and berries and use a cup of juice to make a smoothie.

10 A.M. Take a glass of juice.

Lunch Juice can be used to add variety to the quark-linseed oil cream in desserts

3 P.M. Possibly grape, cherry, pomegranate juice, orange juice.

3:30 P.M. Pineapple or papaya juice.

Juicing Tips

- The cruciferous family, cabbages, kohlrabi, turnips, kale, broccoli and watercress all taste good when pressed with apple and if you add some sort of sharp whole citrus fruits such as orange, the juiced peel increases the antioxidants and tang.
- Tomatoes, peppers, celery and cucumber are great with apple and beet root, try a little garlic and/or onion or even chili peppers.
- Apples, pears, rose-hips or berries are great.
- Carrots and beetroot are great for color and flavor.
- Ginger and lemon are the very best for giving juice a real lift and loads of extra goodness. In a vegetable juice, chilies are surprisingly good.
- Lemon pressed with apple and pear helps keep the juice form going brown.
- "Grasses" which are whole grains of wheat or barley grown to about 7" or 200 mm high are amazing sources of nutrients and ideal for an extra shot of greens in your

juice. Wheat is perhaps richer in nutrients; barley tastes nicer.

- Spinach and Swiss chard make sweeter, less pungent green juices than you might expect.

Juicers

You will need a juicing machine. Whichever juicer you choose, you will be amazed at how good your own home-made fresh juice is. Within reason the more money you spend on a juicer, the better the juice, pressed at cooler temperatures and the more juice is extracted from the pulp – which makes it more cost-effective. Some machines are much easier to clean than others. Budwig prefers Masticating juicer. Omega J-8006 is the best juicer available and it is a masticating type. Juicing on the Budwig Diet is going to be a big part of your life so get a good one (Skelton).

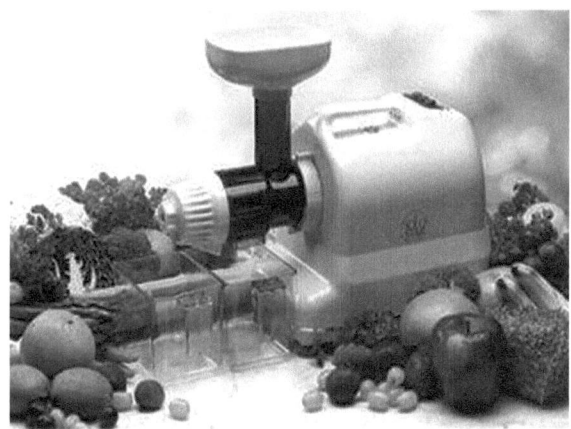

Budwig- Compatible Pain Therapies

Items written in **CAPITALS** are more significant. Foods for managing & healing cancer pain

Flaxseed oil mixed with quark or cottage cheese (Oil Protein Muesli)

Eldi oils (developed by Dr. Johanna Budwig)

A glass of organic sparkling **wine or champagne with linomel.**

Kombucha -

Kombucha is a lightly effervescent fermented drink of sweetened black tea that is used as a functional food. It is produced by fermenting the tea using a symbiotic colony of bacteria and yeast, or "SCOBY". Kombucha contains over 50 different kinds of probiotics, enzymes, amino acids and vitamins. Kombucha is typically produced by placing a culture in a sweetened tea, as sugar is necessary for fermentation. A kombucha scoby (also known as a starter culture, mother etc.) is a necessary component if you wish to make kombucha tea (Schmid, Healing Cancer Naturally).

Cherries

Can help adults maintain an active lifestyle by relieving pain and inflammation. By averting cancer and protecting the nervous system, a diet containing tart cherries may help ensure a future free from debilitating illness. Both sweet and tart cherries are a good source of fiber, vitamin C and potassium. Tart cherries, but not sweet cherries or tart cherry juice, are also an excellent source of vitamin A. Cherries contain a variety of phytochemicals contributing both color and antioxidant activity.

The fruit's dark red color comes from their high content of anthocyanins, which are antioxidants. Strong evidence from several studies has revealed that cherry's anthocyanins offer powerful relief against inflammation and pain (Schmid, Healing Cancer Naturally).

Hydroxycinnamic acid and perillyl alcohol, a phytochemical from the monoterpene family, provide great antioxidant power to cherries.

Preventing and Fighting Cancer - In addition to providing welcome relief from inflammation, antioxidant-rich tart cherries also hold a lot of promise in protecting against cancer.

Supporting Melatonin Levels and Brain Health - Tart cherries are one of the few food sources of melatonin, a chemical released in the body by the pineal gland that is intimately connected with circadian rhythms, or the regulation of the sleep-wake cycle. Melatonin also acts as a powerful antioxidant, providing neuroprotective and immune-modulating effects

Tempeh & FERMENTED SOY products - reduces inflammation

Apple cider vinegar & honey

- One 8 oz glass of cool water
- One cup full of apple cider vinegar
- One Tbsp of organic honey
- Stir well and sip slowly.

Nutritional yeast flakes (Nerve Food): pain stemming from neuritis (inflammation of a nerve) may respond quickly to nutritional yeast, a rich source of B vitamins

Herbs & supplements (organic or wild-crafted)

- ESSIAC
- ALOE VERA
- Maria Treben's herbs
- NONI JUICE
- Mushrooms: MAITAKE (effective in 83% of patients), CORDYCEPS, shiitake & reishi
- DL-PHENYLALANINE (an amino acid)

- Tian Xian paste
- PURPLE CONE FLOWER
- LOBELIA
- Angelica
- Pau d'Arco Tea
- Goldenseal root poultices
- Echinacea (anti-bacterial, anti-viral, anti-parasitic and stimulate lymph flow)
- Mistletoe
- Chaparral
- Turmeric/Curcumin, burdock, ginger - Pain caused by inflammation
- Boswellia Serrata, white willow bark, ginger, green-lipped mussel extract: these anti-inflammatory herbs work against pain triggered by inflammation, inhibit pro-inflammatory mediators, particularly leukotrienes.
- Bromelain/Pineapple
- Oregano Oil (oregano oil can have the same effect on the body as morphine)
- SINUSBUSTER (a nasal spray)
- Hot chili pepper powder in water
- AMYGDALIN/LAETRILE/Vitamin B17

Mind-body approaches to healing cancer pain

- EFT (Emotional Freedom Technique)
- VISUALIZATION, MEDITATION, YOG NIDRA & RELAXATION TECHNIQUES
- Laughter
- Prayer
- EFT
- Tai chi or chi kung (aka taiji or qigong) - not only relieve the pain but lower the fever within fifteen to thirty minutes, sometimes up to two degrees.
- Foot / hand reflexology and massage
- Acupuncture and Reiki
- Bioptron light therapy
- Kinesiology

114

- Biotape
- TENS (Transcutaneous Electrical Nerve Stimulation) Therapy

Detoxification approaches to managing cancer pain

- Alkalizing one's body via fresh juicing and alkaline foods.
- Sodium bicarbonate is also strong alkalizer.
- Coffee enemas and other detox methods
- Dental detox
- Castor oil packs
- Hot baths with Epsom salts
- Water drinking
- Charcoal

Misc.

- Honey packs
- Homeopathic remedies-- particularly Aconitum (1M or 10M dose)
- Exercise
- MSM

Sodium bicarbonate as pain reliever

Sodium bicarbonate is an easily available alkalizer and has been used in many ailments, including cancer. Sodium Bicarbonate has attractive and potent analgesic qualities. Dr. Tullio Simoncini recommends that his cancer patients, undergoing his bicarbonate protocols usually via I.V. administration or orally 1 tsp. of sodium bicarbonate mixed in water per day, for pain control as well as to assist in keeping an alkaline internal environment (Schmid).

Remedy for Bone pain

Bitter apricot kernels may help in the bone pains. You also need zinc (pumpkin seeds) and a make sure you are getting papaya or pineapple every day. Grind the apricot seeds in the coffee grinder with the pumpkin seeds. You need one seed for every 5 kilos of body weight (Schmid).

Healing continues

How long should you take this protocol? If all is well, patient feels better and tumor start to shrink within a 3 or 4 months if he follows treatment religiously and honestly. He may be cured in one or two years. **It is recommended that the Budwig protocol and full diet is followed for at least five years.** Even after that he should maintain healthy eating and life style.

Dr. Budwig has clearly mentioned that if you do not get the desired success do not blame the protocol, rather try to analyze your mistakes and rectify them. Even a minor mistake can unbalance the complete healing process.

Budwig Diet & Protocol - In Brief

This is raw organic diet with lot of Flax oil and Juices. Consume only clean or RO filtered water. To get the best results, proper guidance is strongly recommended. Below are brief guidelines of the Budwig Diet you don't have to consume all the foods on this list. This information is from Dr. Budwig's books.

First thing in the morning – One small glass of sauerkraut juice, preferably raw & homemade. Raw unheated kraut has enzymes, probiotics and vitamins which help the digestive system, metabolize foods & improve immunity.

Just before breakfast - green or herbal tea

Breakfast – First blend 3 Tbsp. Flax oil, 3 Tbsp. milk and a Tsp real honey; then gradually add 6 Tbsp. Quark or Cottage Cheese and blend. Garnish in layers. Add 2 Tbsp freshly ground Flax seeds in a bowl, then add a layer of crushed fresh fruits, then pour oil cheese mixture and put raw nuts on top.

Mid-morning - Homemade vegetable juice (carrots, beets w/lemon or apple, or greens). Homemade carrot is very important cancer-fighters. Carrot juice 4-5 days in a week.

Before Lunch Green or herbal tea.

Lunch - Salad plate (tomato, cucumber, lettuce, radish, cabbage, broccoli, and pepper) with homemade Cottage Cheese and Flax oil **mayo dressing** (prepared by mixing together 2 Tbsp Flax oil, 2 Tbsp milk, 2 Tbsp Cottage Cheese and 1 Tbsp lemon juice, add a variety of herbs making the plate most appealing.

Or use Flax oil and lemon juice / Flax oil and curd dressing.

Lunch - Main Course should be light take early at 12:30. Vegetables/ pulses cooked in water, then flavored with oleolox (Electron butter), spices and herbs possibly with oatmeal, idly, rice (brown) or chapatti etc. Vegetable soups/ sambhar flavored with a little oleolox and nutritional yeast flakes, as side dish for buckwheat, brown rice, millet or potatoes.

Lunch Dessert - Must have 2nd serving of 3 Tbsp. Flax oil and 6 Tbsp. Quark or Cottage Cheese with a little milk and honey, well blended. Add raw fruit, fruit juice, raw nuts, and other flavors you like. You may also refrigerate and serve as ice cream.

Mid-afternoon - 1 Tbsp. freshly ground Flax seed added to 1 glass of pure fruit juice, homemade.

Late afternoon - Enzyme juice - Papaya or pineapple juice, 1 glass.

Dinner also should be light take early at 6:30- Grains alone or grains & beans with vegetables with oleolox, nutritional yeast flakes & spices. Eat **buckwheat at least 4 days in a week.** Grains & beans combined make a complete protein. Vegetables such as spinach, asparagus, broccoli, & cabbage add nutrition and aid absorption.

Late Evening - 1 glass of grape juice (optional) before 10 P.M. if possible.

Linomel Muesli or Oil-Protein Muesli

This should be made fresh and consumed within 15 minutes. It is full of high energy pi-electrons, attract oxygen in the cells and capable of healing cell membranes. It is full of energy-rich omega-3 fats, has power to attract healing photons from sun through resonance. As "Om" is divine word and synonym of God in India. According to Hindu Mythology, the whole universe is located inside "Om", so the name Omkhand has been given to this wonderful recipe in Hindi.

Ingredients

- 3 Tbsp cold pressed organic Flax seed oil (FO)
- 100-125gm (6 Tbsp) Quark or Cottage Cheese (CC)
- 2 Tbsp freshly ground Flax seeds
- 2-3 Tbsp milk
- 1 cup fruits
- ¼ cup dried nuts
- Natural honey
- Flavorings – lemon, apple cider vinegar, cinnamon, pure cacao, natural vanilla, shredded coconut etc.

Recipe

Place 2 tablespoons Linomel or freshly ground Flax seeds in a small bowl. It is covered with raw, crushed or diced seasonal fruits depending on the season. Pour some orange or grape juice over this. Linomel is a brand name and originally created and patented by Budwig. It is a cereal made from cracked Flax Seed, a small amount of honey and a little milk powder.

Then the Quark-Flax seed oil cream is prepared in as follows: First add Flax seed oil, milk and honey and blend briefly with a hand-held immersion electric blender, then gradually add the Quark in smaller portions. Blend till oil and Quark is thoroughly mixed with no separated oil. Then it is seasoned differently everyday with different flavorings such as vanilla, cinnamon or various fruits such as banana, apple, lemon, orange juice, or berries.

Use various fruits such as fresh berries, apple, cherry, orange, banana, papaya, grapes etc. Add other fresh fruit if you like, totaling 1/2 to 1 cup of fruit. Budwig specially advised to use berries like strawberry, blueberry, raspberry, cheery etc. because berries have ellagic acids which are strong cancer fighters.

Add organic raw nuts such as walnuts, almonds, raisins or Brazil nuts. They have sulfurated proteins, omega-3 fats and vitamins. Brazil nut is especially important because a single nut provides you with all of the selenium you need for the day. Selenium is very important to boost immune power. Peanuts are prohibited.

For variety and flavor, try natural vanilla, cinnamon, lemon juice, pure cocoa or shredded coconut.

Once blended in Budwig Cream, Quark and Flax seed oil form a new substance called lipoprotein. Lipoprotein is a water soluble complex. The Quark is rich in the sulfur-containing amino acids, methionine and cysteine. These positively charged amino acids attract the negatively charged electron clouds in fatty acid chains and exhibit a stabilizing effect on the highly unsaturated, otherwise easily oxidized fats. Thus, the amino acids protect the polyunsaturated fatty acids from the Flax seed oil against oxidation which, as a result, are able to enter the human body unchanged and with their full energy potential. The result: they are much more valuable to cells and their membranes. Consequently, one could say that Quark excels as a protector for the polyunsaturated fatty acids.

Sulfur-rich amino acids play a wealth of roles in many vital functions in our bodies. In combination with polyunsaturated fatty acids, they are important partners in regulating the uptake of oxygen and its utilization by the cell. They therefore contribute significantly to a strong immune system, healthy metabolism, and mental vitality. For many generations, people have been getting their omega-3 fatty acids from fish, vegetables, nuts, and seeds. Our health literally depends on the regular consumption of the essential omega-3 and omega-6 fatty acids, alpha-linolenic acid (ALA) and linoleic acid (LA). Our bodies require these fatty acids in order to synthesize their cell membranes as well as for a variety of metabolic processes and heal the cancer and other diseases.

Tips for making the Budwig Mixture
- Follow directions properly! It is important to add things to the mixture in the right order. If you mix them in the wrong order you may lose a lot of the opportunity to convert the oil-soluble omega-3 into water soluble-omega-3.
- Keep the Flax seed oil refrigerated.
- Immersion blender is a must.
- The mixture can be flavored differently every day by adding nuts and fruits preferably organic such as pecans, almonds or walnuts (not peanuts), banana, organic cocoa, shredded coconut, pineapple (fresh) blueberries, raspberries, cinnamon, vanilla or (freshly) squeezed fruit juice.
- Consume immediately for best results.

Prohibitions of Budwig Protocol
- No Sugar, no meat, no eggs, no Butter
- No hydrogenated fat and refined oil
- No soya, corn, peanuts and refined table salt
- No frying, no sautéing, no deep frying
- No preservatives and processed Food
- No microwave, Teflon coated nonstick and aluminum cookware

- No cosmetics, chemicals and pesticides
- No foam mattress and pillow.
- No nylon, polyester or acrylic clothing, only cotton, silk and wool is allowed.
- No Crt. TV and mobile phones
- No leftover food

Elimination or Detoxification

May include (Remember the Mnemonic - M.Sc. Botany)
- Flax oil massage,
- Sun therapy for 20 minutes,
- Coffee enema daily and
- Daily **Soda bicarb bath (40 minutes),** Epsom salt bath, oil pulling, steam bath, sauna bath, liver, colon and kidney cleansing etc.

Energy Therapies (Remember MTV)

Meditation, positive attitude, and deep breathing exercises.

Tumor contract – Tell your tumor that if it grows in size, then you may die, and eventually he also will die. So advise him to become microscopic in size. In return you promise to make some changes in your life so that both of you might live long. If he agrees with your proposal, sign a contract with him immediately.

Visualization – is the most important tool to tap into the power of your imagination to help heal cancer. Remain tuned to your healthy and happy future.

Important and must do therapies with Budwig

- Dandelion root 1 Tsp once a day
- Black seed oil 1 Tsp twice a day
- Bitter apricot kernels 13 seeds with a Tsp pumpkin seeds
- Essiac tea 60ml per day
- Brazil nuts a nut a day
- Cap Nano Curcumin 1 cap thrice a day
- Nutritional yeast flakes/powder 1 Tbsp a day

Skin

The skin is the largest organ of the body, with a total area of about 20 square feet. The skin protects us from microbes and external pollutants, helps regulate body temperature, and permits the sensations of touch, heat, and cold.

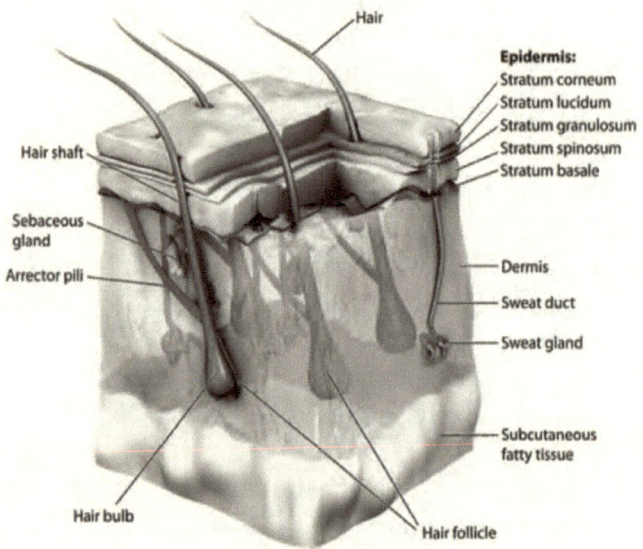

Skin has three layers:

1) **The epidermis on the outside.** This is made from layers of cells with a basal layer, which is always forming new cells through cell division. The new cells gradually move towards the surface, which takes 1-2 months. As they move up they gradually die, become flattened and develop keratin and the outermost layer of flat dead cells is being continually worn away by friction. The keratin and oil from the sebaceous glands help to make the skin waterproof.

2) **The dermis is the inner layer.** The tissues and structures found in the dermis are given below.

- **Elastic fibers** – make the skin resilient.
- **Capillaries** – are tiny blood vessels.
- **Muscle fibers** – to move the position of the hairs.
- **Sensory cells** – to sense touch, pressure, heat, cold and pain.
- **Nerve fibers** – to activate muscles and glands and relay messages from the sensory cells to the brain.
- **Pigment cells which produce Melanin** – a very dark pigment.
- **Sweat glands** which open onto the surface as pores
- **Hair follicles** – pits in the epidermis in which hairs grow.
- **Sebaceous glands** – produce oil to keep hair follicle free from dust and bacteria, and to help to waterproof the skin.
- **There is a layer of fat underneath** and in the lower regions of the dermis. The thickness of this layer varies, depending on the place in the body and from person to person. A store of fat is useful to the body as insulation and it can be used for energy when the intake of nutrients is insufficient.

3) **Connective tissue** – packs and binds the other structures in the skin.

Flaxseed – Skin Healer

If you want one word solution to all your skin, hair and nail problems, my answer is Omega-3 Fats. Free radicals steal electrons from collagen cells in your skin, as a result fine lines are formed in skin which gradually lead to age spots, wrinkles and sagging of skin. Skin becomes dry and looks older. This is ageing of skin.

Omega-3 Key to Healthy skin

Omega-3 fats and Lignans present in flax protect collagen cells and make your skin fair, soft, spotless and charming. Flaxseed is an ultimate edible cosmetic, which glows your skin from inside. It keeps you young and attractive.

Flaxseed – Skin's best friend

According to Dr. Jeffrey Benabio, dermatologist, Flax protects your skin in two ways. First, everyday irritants are kept from entering skin pores. Secondly, water is locked into your skin when you apply flaxseed oil directly onto your skin. Improving your skin's moisture level can minimize the appearance of wrinkles.

Flaxseed - heals all skin ailments

Flax is full of Omega-3 fats which are Anti-inflammatory and heal inflamed red and itchy skin. These fats also cures skin spots, rashes, ulcers, boils, pimples due to allergy and infection. This way flax treats rosacea, acne, eczema, dandruff, psoriasis and even skin tumors.

Wound healing – Flax oil has been shown to aid in wound healing as well. Wounds heal and recover faster. Possibility of large scar and keloid formation is much less. There is even some evidence that flax oil might protect against ultraviolet light (sun) damage and can help protect you against skin cancer.

Hair

HAIR ANATOMY

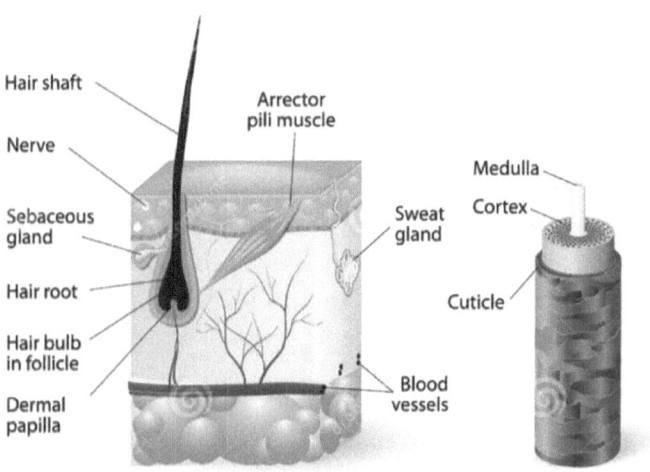

The hair shaft has three layers. Cuticle is the outer transparent layers and gives a shiny appearance to hair. Medulla is the innermost layer composed of large cells. Cortex is the black, thick and hard layer between cuticle and medulla. This contains pigment and keratin.

The root of hair is situated in the skin (epidermis) of scalp. A pouch like structure called follicle surrounds the hair root. Papilla is a large structure at the base of the hair follicle. The papilla is made up mainly of connective tissue and a capillary loop.

Around the papilla is the Matrix, a collection of cells often interspersed with the pigment-producing cells, melanocytes.

Capillaries and nerve fibers indent this bulb. The cells in the center of bulb divide. The newly divided hair cells push the previous cells up. The cells, which move upwards, die slowly forming hard hair shaft.

Each hair grows approximately at the rate of 1 cm per month. This growth continues for 2-6 years. When the hair attains full growth it resets for 2-3 months and is later shed. A new hair starts growing in its place. Thus at any given point of time 10 percent of the total hair on our scalp is in a resting phase and 90 percent of the hair is in growth phase.

Keratin – Building block of Hair

Hair is composed primarily of hard fibrous proteins (88%) known as keratin. It is made in cells of Follicle called keratinocytes, some of these make outer and inner epithelium of follicle, remaining elongate and become shaft of hair. As soon as keratinocyte is filled with keratin, it becomes dead. This way after the growth of 0.5 mm hair becomes mature, dead and does not receive any nutrition afterwards.

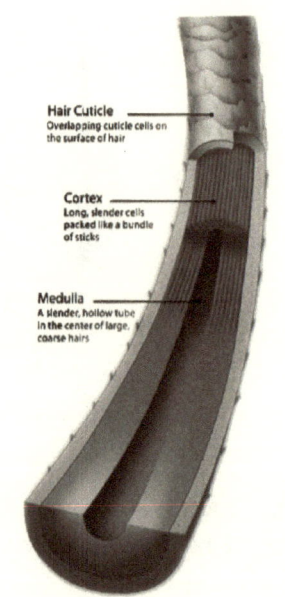

Hair Cuticle
Overlapping cuticle cells on the surface of hair

Cortex
Long, slender cells packed like a bundle of sticks

Medulla
A slender, hollow tube in the center of large, coarse hairs

Sebum - Natural oil of hair and skin

Fats play very important role for strength and shining of hair, even though quantity of fat is just 3%. There are sebaceous glands near hair follicle which produce sebum. It is a mixture of triglycerides, wax and squalene which provide protective coating for skin and hair. And makes skin elastic and shining.

Melanin - Natural Color of skin and hair

Melanocyte cells in the follicle produce natural color pigment Melanin. Keratinocytes take this pigment to give natural color to the hair. There are two main pigments found in human hair: Eumelanin which gives color to brown or black hair and is dark pigment. Pheomelanin is what produces the blonde or red hair.

Flaxseed - Secret of silky hair

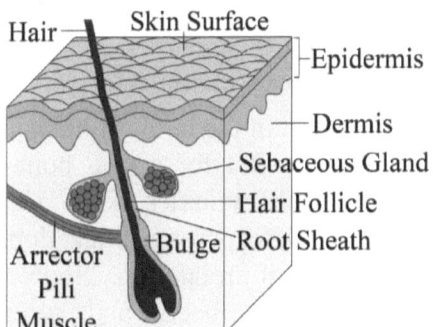

Flax is very miraculous for hair. It is a secret of long, thick, shining, strong and healthy hair. Flax prevent/ reverses premature graying of hair. Lignan has antifungal properties, so regular flax eaters never develop Dandruff.

Essential Nutrients for Hair

Omega-3 Fats - Omega-3 fats are basic building block required to make anti-inflammatory hormones and prostaglandins. They are very essential for healthy scalp skin and sebum production.

Protein – A deficiency can cause you to lose shine and definition, interfere with your moisture levels and ultimately result in stunted hair growth. Sources are whole grains, nuts, beans and legumes, eggs, lean meats, poultry

Vitamin A - Antioxidant that helps produce healthy sebum in the scalp. It's also beneficial to hair follicles, as it keeps the hair root lubricated. Food sources are fish liver oil, liver, meat, milk, cheese, eggs, spinach, broccoli, green leafy vegetables, cabbage, carrots, and orange vegetables, apricots and peaches.

Vitamin B Complex - A deficiency of Vitamin B group may cause hair loss, excessive oil reproduction and premature graying.

Eating things like whole grains, beans and lentils, potatoes and bananas will aid with restoring those deficiencies.

Vitamin C - is what we count on for growth and cell repair. A deficiency can stunt length your hair and interfere with your scalp's circulation and healing abilities. Oranges, papaya, grapefruit, cauliflower and asparagus can help restore depleted levels of Vitamin C.

Vitamin E - plays an important role in proper scalp circulation and the oil levels of your hair strands. A deficiency may cause overly dry, brittle hair and ultimately result in hair loss. Avocados, nuts like almonds and hazelnuts, tomatoes and beets into your diet will help you maintain proper Vitamin E levels.

Silica – Balances calcium and magnesium in the body. It helps to deposit phosphorus in the bones and is vital for strong bones. Silica helps in collagen formation, heals wrinkles, keep skin moist, radiant and young. It is essential for strong, thick, long and lustrous hair. It is also required for nail production. Sources are oatmeal, wheat, rice, millet, onion, beets and green vegetables.

Zinc, selenium manganese and copper – are very important minerals for healthy skin, hair and nails. Deficiency leads to eczema, hair loss and other problems. Zinc reduces levels of DHT which is a major cause of male baldness. Zinc is an anti-oxidant, protects hair Follicle, helps in DNA and RNA production, Reproduction, Growth, Eye and Thyroid Gland functioning. Copper is Anti-inflammatory and is required for healing of wound and wrinkles. It is vital for rich, black and long hair.

Sources of minerals

- Zinc - Spinach, flax, mushrooms, butter, whole grains, legumes, egg, dry fruits etc.
- Selenium – Brazil nut, walnuts, sesame, flax, wheat, soy bean, meat, fish and eggs.
- Copper – Sesame, flax, cocoa, cashew nut, pumpkin and sun flower seeds.

- Manganese – Cloves, red chilies, flax, sesame, dry fruits, cocoa, pumpkin and sun flower seeds.

Biotin – Vitamin of Hair

Biotin or vitamin B7 or vitamin H, supporting the growth of healthy hair, biotin has a direct role in the formation of keratin. It is often prescribed as a treatment for healing dry scalps, treating brittle fingernails and for re-activating hair growth in people experiencing hair loss. It is composed of a ureido ring fused with a tetrahydrothiophene ring. Biotin is a coenzyme for carboxylase enzymes, involved in the synthesis of fatty acids, isoleucine, and valine, and in gluconeogenesis.

It helps cell growth, citric acid cycle, and transport of carbon dioxyde. Sources of biotin are carrot, almonds, walnuts, egg, milk, strawberry, halibut fish, onion, cucumber and cauliflower.

Nail – The Barometer of your health

Our nails are barometer of our general well-being and often act as indicators of health problems elsewhere in the body. It shows status of blood circulation in fingers. Examination of nails help doctor to identify many illnesses or nutrient deficiencies.

Anatomy of Nail

Basically nail is part of skin on the back of finger and toes. And is made of hard and thick protein called keratin. On three sides it is surrounded by skin folds. The hard and visible part of 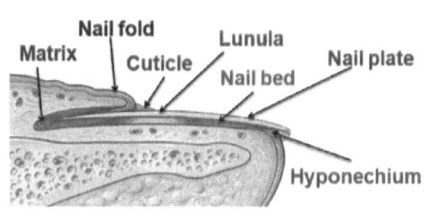 nail is called nail plate. Nail plate is situated and fused over nail bed. The light semicircular proximal part of nail plate is called Lunula. The tissue joining Fold of skin and lunula is called

Aponechium or cuticle. Nail grows from matrix situated under the nail cuticle. Nail grows about 0.1 mm in a day.

Nutrients for healthy nails

For making and repair of nails Vitamin B group, Biotin, Calcium, Zinc, Copper, Protein and Omega-3 fats are very important. Their deficiency leads to dry, weak and brittle nails. Vitamin-B deficiency, especially biotin, will

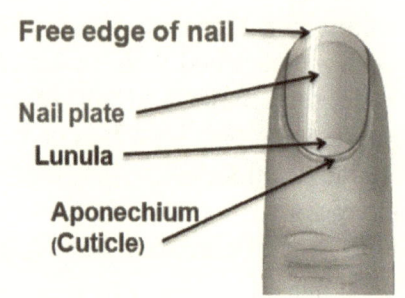

Free edge of nail →
Nail plate →
Lunula →
Aponechium (Cuticle) →

produce ridges along the bed of the nail. Lack of iron causes concave and deformed nails.

Flaxseed for Healthy nail

Luckily Flaxseed contains almost all of these nutrients so regular consumption of flaxseed remodels nails and leads to healthy strong, beautiful, pink and spotless nails. Though it does not contain Biotin.

Flaxseed and Osteoarthritis

Arthritis is an inflammation of a joint or joints in the body. One of the most common types of arthritis is osteoarthritis or "degenerative arthritis." Often described as ageing disease or "wear and tear" arthritis, it affects more than 15 million Americans.

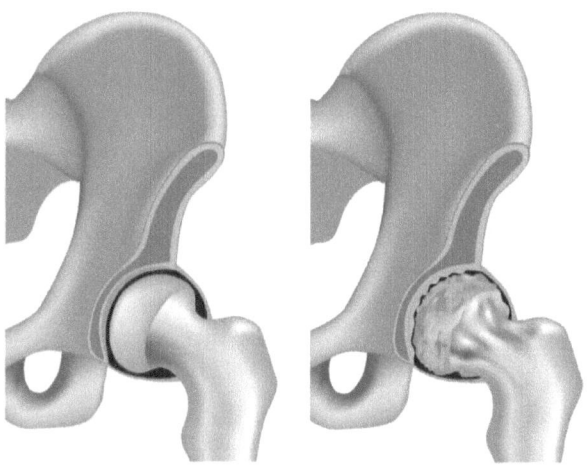

Healthy hip joint   Osteoarthritis

Osteoarthritis follows the breakdown of cartilage in a joint, eventually leading to abnormal bone changes. The role of joints is to provide flexibility, stability, support and protection to the skeleton, allowing movement of limbs and the entire body. Cartilage assists in these functions by coating the ends of the bones. In the early stages of osteoarthritis, the surface of the cartilage becomes swollen, forming tiny crevasses which hinder normal joint functioning. Inflammation may also occur in the synovium, a fluid-filled sac that surrounds the joint and provides nutrients and oxygen to the joint components. As the cartilage loses elasticity, it becomes vulnerable to further damage from repetitive use, which can cause a great deal of pain and swelling. In advanced cases, there is a complete loss of cartilage cushion between the joint and bone, which ultimately limits joint mobility. The joints most commonly affected are the knees, hips, spine, hands and toes.

Symptoms of osteoarthritis

- Pain in the affected joint after repeated use, especially later in the day.
- Swelling, pain and stiffness after long periods of inactivity, such as waking in the morning, that subsides with movement and activity.
- Continuous pain, even at rest, is a symptom of advanced osteoarthritis, when there is total loss of cartilage.
- In osteoarthritis of the spine, pain can occur in the neck or lower back. If bony spurs develop, the nerves exiting from the spine can be irritated, causing numbness, tingling and severe pain in the back or limbs. Osteoarthritis in the fingers can result in hard bony enlargements, and bunions can form at the base of the big toe if the feet are affected.
- The degree of symptoms varies among individuals. Some people become completely debilitated, while others may experience few symptoms despite the severity of their condition. Symptoms may also be intermittent, and some individuals go for long periods of time relatively symptom-free.

Lifestyle Changes

- **Lose weight** if you are overweight - it can alleviate excess mechanical stress on the affected joints.
- **Avoid intense activities** that injure or strain the joint cartilage.
- **Exercise -** This can actually be beneficial as long as it is performed at a level that does not stress the affected joints. Strengthening surrounding muscles will support and protect the joint, and physical activity helps improve

and maintain joint mobility and aids weight-reduction efforts. The safest activities are swimming, stationary cycling and light weight training - which put little stress on the joints.

Dietary changes

- **Flaxseed** - Studies show that people who suffer from arthritis may benefit by consumption of omega 3 fatty acids which are found in flax seed oil. Nutrients found in flax seed oil contain anti-inflammatory agents, which can help quell the inflammation of joints that leads to aches and pains helping reduce the risk of arthritis.
- **Ginger and Turmeric** - Research has shown that the ginger and turmeric may help reduce inflammation. Regularly use ginger and turmeric. Ginger tea is a good example. Foods rich in antioxidants - plentifully found in most vegetables and fruit - may help reduce tissue damage from inflammation.

Supplements

- **Glucosamine sulfate** - Glucosamine sulfate provides the joints with the building blocks they need to help repair the natural wear on cartilage caused by everyday activities. Specifically, glucosamine sulfate provides the raw material needed by the body to manufacture a mucopolysaccharide (called glycosaminoglycan) found in cartilage. Supplemental sources are derived from shellfish. Taken in supplement form, glucosamine may help improve the maintenance of healthy cartilage with an enhanced deposition of glycosaminoglycan.
- **Chondroitin** - Chondroitin protects the cartilage and attracts fluids that give the tissue its shock absorbing quality.
- **Evening primrose oil** - A source of gamma-linolenic acid (GLA) which may help maintain healthy joints by modifying inflammation.

- **Herbs and spices** - Ginger, holy basil, turmeric, green tea, rosemary and bosvelia serrata all have naturally occurring anti-inflammatory compounds known as COX-2 inhibitors.
- **Flaxseed Oil -** which have been shown in studies to help maintain bone health and flexibility.

Flax– Good for athletes as well as weight watchers !!!

How is it possible that high-quality cold-pressed flaxseed oil can benefit both top performance athletes to build their lean muscles and obese people who want to get rid of fat deposited in their body? Strange, but it is true. The answer lies in the multiple benefits of alpha-linolenic acid (ALA), found in flaxseed oil in abundance.

Flaxseed oil - great energy source - First, flaxseed oil is a great energy source, especially for endurance athletes and those who burn lots of calories during rigorous workouts. The body does not store enough glycogen to fulfill this energy need. Although the brain uses sugar as its main energy source, the rest of the body uses fat, and flaxseed fatty acids provide clean-burning fuel for tough training routines without disturbing blood sugar level the way refined carbohydrates do.

Produce anti-inflammatory molecules Vigorous exercise puts great stress on muscles, tendons, and joint tissues. Fortunately, the local hormones (prostaglandins) synthesized from omega-3 fatty acids (such as EPA produced from ALA) on cell membranes are anti-inflammatory. Therefore, the tendency for tissue to become inflamed after exercise is vastly reduced. This benefit shortens recovery time and allows athletes to stay at their performance peak longer.

Make healthy membranes for muscle repair - Vigorous exercise often causes micro-tears in muscles. Protein helps repair muscle cells and essential fatty acids are most important to build cell, nuclear, and mitochondrial membranes that help to remodel and refurbish muscle and connective tissues.

Minimized deposit of subcutaneous fats - For body builders trying to create muscle mass that they want to be seen, the last thing they need is an energy source that will deposit body fat over muscles. This will hide the muscle they have worked so hard to build. Research has demonstrated that animal fats in the diet cause more storage of depot fat on the body than vegetable fats. And of the vegetable fats, ALA sources, such as flaxseed oil, cause the least amount of new fat storage compared to the omega-6 sources, such as corn, sunflower, or safflower oils.

What does all of this mean for **athletes and bodybuilders?**

- Reduced Body fat
- Enhanced Performance
- Shortened recovery time
- Good source of energy
- Reduced muscle soreness
- Increased utilization of oxygen
- Increased utilization of other nutrients
- Overall better health

and what do all of these lead to?   MORE MUSCLE!

The biggest and more publicly discussed example of the benefits of flaxseed oil for athletic performance is preparing Hilary Swank for her role as a boxer in Clint Eastwood's famous film, Million Dollar Baby. A renowned Canadian trainer, Grant Roberts, who owns many gyms in the U.S. and Canada, was given this job. He had the responsibility of adding 10 pounds of lean muscle to her already lean physique in just nine weeks. To everybody's surprise, Mr. Roberts's and Swank's hard work added more than 20 pounds of muscle in that time. How could this be achieved?

An intense weight-training program and lots of practice honing her boxing skills, he put her on a daily 4,000 calorie diet. Half of those calories were in the form of high-protein. One quarter (1000 calorie) of her diet was in the form of flaxseed oil (8 or 9 tablespoons oil in a day). The choice of flaxseed oil was a smart decision based on his hard-earned experience. The film was a big hit and snatched four Oscar awards.

According to Mr. Roberts, nutrition represents 60% to 70% of the effective input to building lean muscle mass. The remaining 30% to 40% of positive results arise from a wisely planned exercise routine. Thus, there is no substitute for proper nutrition in athletics, and too few coaches and trainers tell this wisdom to their clients.

So why is a top personal trainer like Grant Roberts so keen on using flaxseed oil? In addition to optimal hydration, energy source, flaxseed oil can give a winning shape to the professional or amateur athlete. The benefits of flax oil are wide ranging.

Flaxseed has received an overwhelming response from the athletic and bodybuilding community. An article entitled "Best of the Best", published in the bodybuilding and health enthusiast magazine Muscle Media 2000, claims flaxseed as "the hottest idea in bodybuilding" and "a surprising new category of bodybuilding supplement." Mr. Dan Duchene in his column "Ask the Guru", also writing for Muscle Media 2000, and ranked flaxseed as the number one bodybuilding supplement compared to all other available products.

How does flaxseed oil helps lose Weight

So how do all these benefits of flaxseed oil help to lose weight? First we need to come out of the fat phobia that has been infused in our mind by American media for years. Scientific researchers are now investigating the importance of the type of fat, rather than the absolute quantity of fat, we consume. There are good fats and bad fats. Bad fat is a major risk factor in chronic diseases, while good fats are essential and very important for us. This also applies to obesity and weight management.

Americans normally consume more omega-6 laden animal fats, put more depot fat on the body than natural vegetable oils. And among the vegetable oils, ALA sources, such as flaxseed oil, put the least amount of depot fat on the body. Recent research shows that omega-3 fatty acids actually help to enhance the body metabolism to increase thermogenesis, the generation of body heat to burn off excess calories.

Adding flaxseed to your diet

Flaxseed adds a pleasant, nutty taste to foods. You can buy raw Flaxseed, already ground Flax meal, and Flaxseed Oil. Here are some ways to use flaxseed.

- Whole flaxseeds add color and crunch to foods. You can sprinkle flaxseed powder on top of home baking or mix them into a dough.
- Grinding whole seeds breaks their tough outer skin, creating a light-colored powder. Milled flaxseed is sold in a vacuum packs or you can prepare it yourself in a coffee grinder. Sprinkle milled flaxseed on cereal or add it to doughs, batters, casseroles and other cooked foods.
- **Flaxseed oil** is sold in bottles. It is a **sun shine** in a bottle. Pour flaxseed oil on fresh salads. Flaxseed oil provides ALA but no fiber or lignans. Flaxseed oil is also available in gel capsules and sold as a dietary supplement.
- Omega-3 enriched eggs contain extra omega-3 fatty acids from flaxseed fed to hens. You can use omega-3 eggs wherever you would use regular eggs – there's no taste difference, only nutrition enrichment. If eaten on a regular basis, omega-3 enriched eggs make a substantial contribution to your need for omega-3 fatty acids. The caloric value and protein content of omega-3 enriched eggs are similar to that of regular eggs.
- Omega-3 enriched foods, such as yogurt and milk, may contain flaxseed oil, while flaxseed baked goods, such as breads, can include milled or whole flaxseed.
- Whole flaxseeds do not break down in the digestive system. If you consume them whole, chew them thoroughly. Even then, many may not have broken down and will pass through the digestive system without being

absorbed. Still, they offer the benefits of fiber by cleansing the intestinal tract. Store flaxseed meal in the refrigerator.

- Be sure to drink plenty of water when consuming flaxseeds or the flaxseed meal because flax tends to absorb large quantities of liquid during the digestion process.
- Raw is the only way to consume flax oil. Do not use flax oil for cooking. When polyunsaturated oils such as flaxseed oil are subjected to high heat, their chemical make-up is converted to unhealthful lipid peroxides.

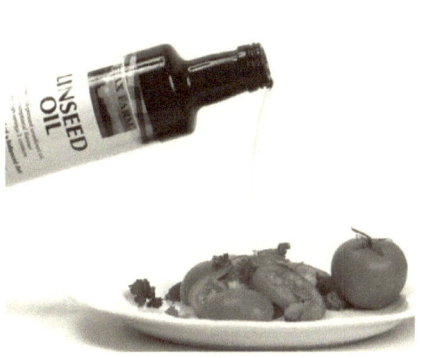

How much flax to eat

- Like any high fiber food, flaxseed may upset your digestion if you add too much, too quickly. Healthy people should consume 15-20 g (2-3 Tbsp.) of milled flaxseed as part of a balanced diet.
- **For individuals at risk of developing, or who have heart disease, a daily intake of 30-40g (5 Tbsp.) of milled flaxseed is recommended by Health Department of Canada. Never buy roasted flax seeds.**

Storing Flaxseed

You can store whole flaxseed, which is clean, dry and of good quality, at room temperature for up to a year.

To keep flaxseed fresh, you should grind it when you need it. You can keep milled flaxseed refrigerated in an airtight, opaque container for up to 30 days, but it is not recommended.

Fat or Oil Substitution Instructions

Use a 3:1 ratio when substituting flaxseed for oil in a recipe. For example, 3 tablespoons of milled flaxseed can replace 1 tablespoon of butter, margarine, shortening or vegetable oil.

Egg Substitution Instructions:

For every egg being replaced, mix 1 tablespoon milled flaxseed with 3 tablespoons water in a small bowl and let sit for one or two minutes. The mixture will become gel-like. Add to your recipe as you would an egg.

Omega-3

Apple Cider Vinaigrette

Ingredients:
- 4 Tbsp Flaxseed Oil
- 2 Tbsp Apple Cider Vinegar
- 1 Clove of Garlic (pressed)
- Fresh herbs of your choice finely chopped (cilantro, basil, parsley, etc.)

Preparation
Combine all the ingredients together and either mix all manually, or use a handheld blender and blend together.

Lemon Vinaigrette

Ingredients:
- 4 Tbsp Flaxseed Oil
- 2 Tbsp Fresh Lemon Juice
- 1 Clove of Garlic (crushed)
- Fresh herbs of your choice finely chopped (cilantro, basil, parsley etc.)

Preparation

Combine all the ingredients together and either mix all manually, or use a handheld blender and blend together.

Balsamic Vinaigrette

Ingredients:

- 1 1/4 t. salt
- 1/4 t. dry mustard
- 4 to 5 cloves garlic, minced
- 1/2 C. (120 ml) flax oil
- 1/2 C. (120 ml) balsamic vinegar
- 1/4 C. (60 ml) lemon juice
- 1/4 C. (60 ml) water

Preparation

Combine all ingredients in a jar and shake well. Keep refrigerated and shake well before each use. Use within 2 weeks. For a creamier alternative, combine all ingredients in a blender, and blend on high speed until well combined and smooth.

Sprouting flaxseeds

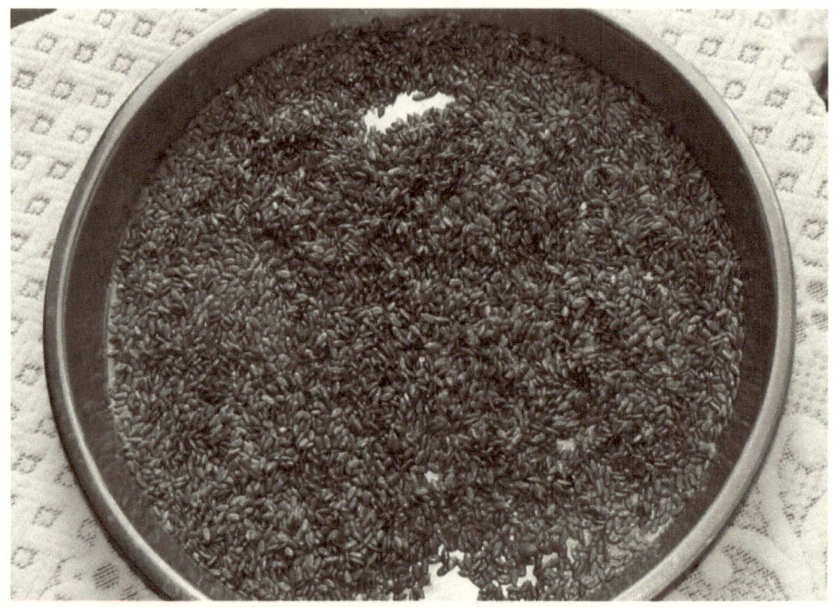

Making sprouts of flaxseeds is so easy you won't believe it! They just can't be done any other way... otherwise these become too gelatinous and spoil. Just put the seeds directly on a steel plate and watch them grow!

You need the following items.

- Two large stainless steel plates
- Water spray bottle
- Flaxseeds approx 100 grams

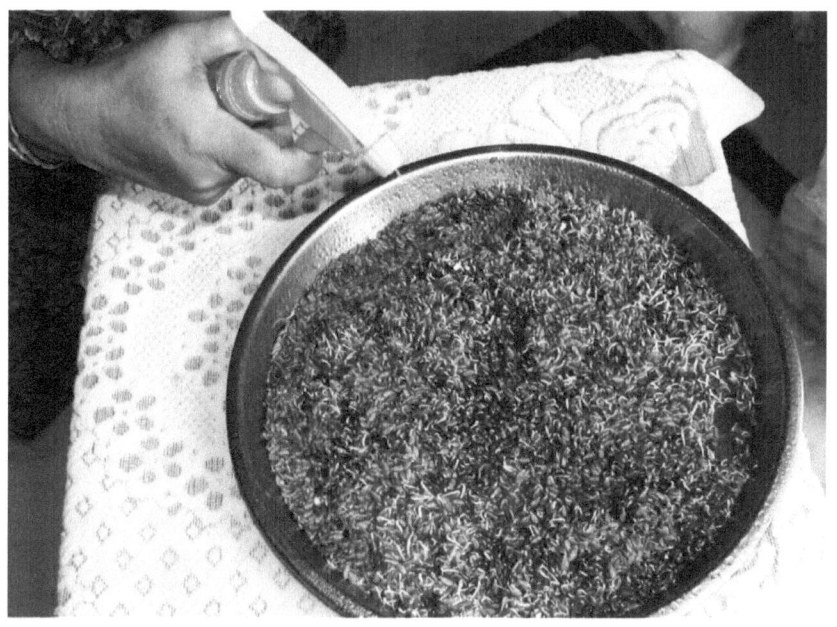

Procedure – Take a stainless steel plate and spread the flaxseeds evenly in this plate. Then fill RO water in the spray bottle. Nicely spray water over flaxseeds. Cover this plate with another steel plate and keep these on a table. After 15 minutes remove the cover plate and check the flaxseeds in the bottom plate. You will see that flaxseeds have absorbed all the water and are almost dry. Spray the water over flaxseeds again, cover and keep upon the table. In the beginning check the flaxseeds frequently and spray water if desired. Afterwards it is enough to check every 3-4 hours in a day. The basic idea is that you give controlled amount of moisture to the seeds. If you pour more water, the soluble fiber mucilage swells up and become gelatinous. If everything is fine, you will get beautiful flaxseed sprouts on third day. Sprouts may have approx. 1 cm. long white and shining roots. We have tried many procedures, but this is the best procedure to make wonderful flax sprouts.

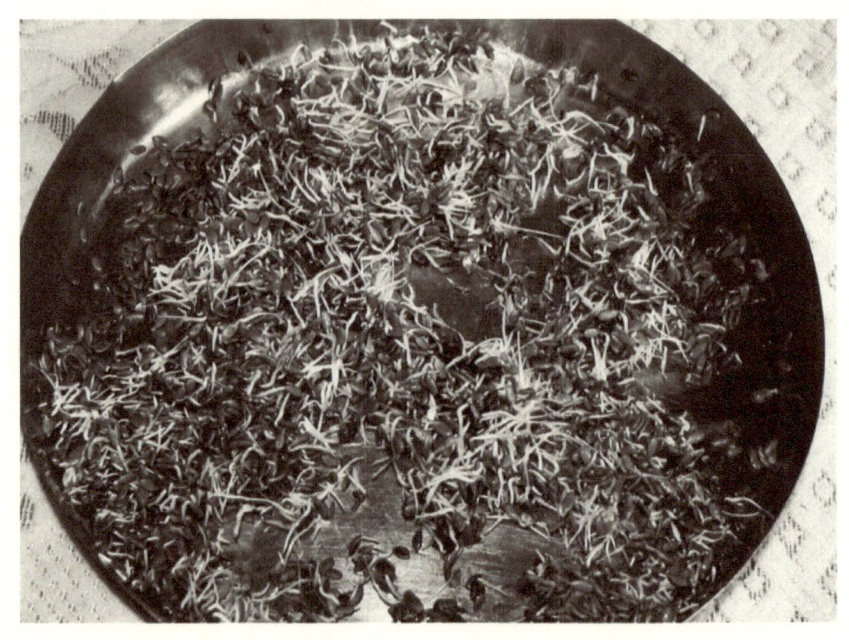

Testimonials and Letters

Dr. O.P.Tandon

Dr. O.P.Tandon is a friend of mine and lives in Ajmer. He is retired Principal of College and his age is 76 years. He always appreciates my work. He promotes and eats flaxseeds for good health. On Jan 4, 2013, he called me to wish New Year. **He also told me with full confidence that his scalp hair is absolutely turned black.** I also did not be believe that a man can regain his black hair at the age of 76, but is true. Wow!

Mrs. Dessa

In Delhi I met a lady who told an interesting story about miracles of awesome Flax. Before a year or so, she had pain in her right breast. She consulted her doctor. He did her Mamogram. After reviewing the scan he told her that cause of her pain is calcifications in the breast tissue that will subside with some medicines. There nothing to worry.

She took the medicines for 6 months but there was no relief in pain. Then she started to eat flaxseeds and her pain vanished absolutely in just 14 days. Awesome Flax!

Jai Prakash Narayan

Respected Dr. O.P.Verma,

Regards

I am very happy to write this letter. I read your article about flaxseeds in Nirogdham magazine in Jan, 2010. I was highly impressed by this article. I immediately started eating 30 grams of flaxseed daily. And within few days I was full of vital energy.

Before I was suffering from many health problems, but today I am perfectly healthy. I feel and enjoy youth of 25 years at my age of 53 years. It looks as if a new wave of youth, bliss and energy is flowing in my body. Now you are my Guru, my master. I am highly impressed by you. Your article has entirely changed my life. I want to meet you in person as soon as possible. I don't have words to explain my joy and happiness. Now I dream to live for 100 years.

I never thought that this will happen. Now I am telling everybody to use Flaxseed and remain healthy. Flaxseed is a fountain of youth and health. I have given photocopies of your great article to hundreds of people. God bless you, Sir.

Yours only,

Jai Prakash Narayan Shrivastava
Rly. Qtr. No. 568/B
TRS colony Gomoh
Dist – Dhanbad (Jharkhand) Pin – 828401
Date 02/02/11

Dheeraj Sharma

From
Anonymous
Kashipur, Uttrakhand

Respected Dr. O.P.Verma,

I am AIDS patient since a few years. I was taking treatment. But I suffered from side effects of the drugs and developed jaundice. My platelet count became low. Then my wife read your article. You advised 3 tbsp flaxseed oil with cottage cheese for me. I started your treatment. I also consumed coconut oil as you told my wife. This treatment gave a lot of benefits. My CD count increased from 210 to 538 in just 4 months. It is very good. I am not disclosing my real name.

Anonymous

Anil Paul

Anil Paul
Jagatpura, Jaipur Rajasthan
Mobile No# 9214044523

My wife was Myopic and was wearing glasses since 35 years. She also suffers from chronic flu since many years. Every day she used to take anti-allergic tablet. Then we started eating flaxseed after meeting you. After 6 months a miracle happened. Her chronic flu was absolutely cured and vision improved. No glasses were needed any more. We still eat flaxseeds daily. We are highly obliged by you.

Thanks.

Anil Paul

Keshavram Bhakt

Respected Dr. O.P.Verma,

Regards.

Your article "Awesome Flax" was published in Srijankarm, Norogdham, Sehat, Yog Sandesh, Aha! Zindagi, Pension Chintan and many other magazines in last one and half years. I read it many times, and thought that I must consume this wonder seed, because I was highly impressed by your article.

I started to eat flaxseed in April, 2010. Today in January, 2011 my Constipation is completely cured. Hemorrhoids have become very small and rudimentary. Sugar control is smooth. I have become very active, positive, and very energetic. My appetite is increased and I have sound sleep. My skin is shining. People say I look much younger to my age (69 years). Flaxseed is really a super star anti-ageing food, as you wrote in your article. I am highly thankful to you for giving such a healthy food to community.

Now I want to spread this knowledge to my friend and countrymen. I shall work for awareness of flaxseed till my death.

I am distributing brochures of flaxseed given by you. I have written at least 1000 long letters to my friends and relatives to spread this awareness.

Here I want to give example of my friend Rohit Kumar. He is a patient of Diabetes and Blood Pressure with Kidney problem. He had edema in both feet. He was taking treatment from a big Hospital. I told him to take Flaxseeds. Now he is much better may be 90%.

Thank you very much for this great service for the society. I invite you to Dhamtari for a flaxseed seminar.

Keshavram Bhakt
Retired Teacher Dhamtari
Mobile 09479205714
Date 6.1.2011

Raman A Patel

Motivated by Dr. O.P.Verma's article on flaxseed in Yog Sandesh I started taking flaxseed regularly since September, 11. 40 gms. of freshly ground lightly roasted flaxseed mixed thoroughly with curds. Dr. Verma had kindly sent me analysis of composition of flaxseeds. It is full of high quality proteins, carbohydrates, vitamins and minerals and above all omega-3. For us vegetarians it is a rich source of omega-3 since it contains 18% omega-3. Since it contains almost all the nutrients a human body and brain needs I consumed this as my break-fast. As a result I felt full till lunch time at about 1:00 0'clock.

It sprite of my age which is 80 years I found astonishing results to say the least.

I have been facing prostate gland enlargement problems for the last few years - frequent urination and loss of control resulting in spoiling clothes. The frequency of urination was once every hour during the nights. I have not taken any allopathic medicine for this problem. Since last two weeks I wake up for urination once in two to three hours and I have regained control.

From my childhood I have suffered from dysentery and constipation. Dysentery I got relief from by urine therapy but constipation persisted. Due to high fiber content in flaxseed. I have great relief in constipation only a sufferer will know how big relief this is!!!

This is only an interim report. I hope to report back in 3 month time about high blood pressure and blood circulation.

Raman A Patel, Yoga Teacher
Mumbai 400057
Date: 12.12.11

Prakash Jain - Flax cured his Arthritis

One of my friends Dr. Manohar Bhandari was posted in Medial College, Jabalpur as Senior Professor before two years. One day he visited a famous Pisanhari Jain Temple situated on a hill top, about 5 Kms from Jabalpur on Jabalpur Nagpur highway. The height of hill is approx. 300 feet. To reach the temple you have to climb 400 steps. The cashier of the temple Mr. Prakash Jain was suffering from Osteoarthritis in both knees. He was taking lot of medicines for pain costing around Rs. 1500/-. For his daily routine he had to go up and down two or three times. It was really very difficult for him to climb the steps of the temple. He asked Dr. Bhandari if he can do something for his joint problem. As Dr. Bhandari was aware about miracles of flaxseed, he advised Prakash to consume 30 grams of Flaxseeds daily.

After one and months Dr. Bhandari again visited Pisanhari Temple. This time Mr. Prakash was very happy and thanked a lot for advising flaxseed. He told that his pain is almost gone and medicines are not needed. He can go to temple three times without any problem.

Achala Kalra

I am regular reader of Nirogdham and I live in Abohar Punjab. I suffer from Osteoarthritis of both knees. Our house is very big. I have lot of pain in my knees. Even walking in the house is a problem. I also had difficulty in going upstairs. Dr. has advised for Joint Replacement Surgery. Then I read flaxseed article by Flax Guru Dr. O.P.Verma in Nirogdham. He has suggested that flaxseed is very miraculous for joint problems. So I preferred to eat Flaxseeds. Some of my friends told me that flaxseed is a useless food and will not do any good. But I did not listen and continued using Flaxseed.

After 4-5 months I got relief in my pain. Now I can easily walk in my house. I can also go for evening walk. Flax is really a superstar food.

Achla Kalra
Phone 1634 - 232932
Street No. 7 Chook No. 1, Old Suraj Nagri
ABOHAR – 152116 (Panjab)

Ravi Kant Prasad

Respected Dr. O.P.Verma,

Regards.

I happily admit that I am able to treat my Diabetes successfully under your guidance. In September, 2008 my Blood Sugar was F 265 and PP 450 mg. I took medicines for few months, but afterwards I became irregular in taking medicines and my Blood Sugar shoot up to F 298 and PP 490 mg. Then somebody told me to consult Flax Guru. And I came to you.

You advised me to mix Flaxseeds in my homemade bread (Chapatti) morning as well as evening. You also changed my cooking oil. You suggested doing evening walk, consuming Chromium, Shilajit, pinch of cinnamon and 2 tbsp cold pressed flaxseed oil. I followed all your suggestions. After 2 months my Blood Sugar was F 108 and PP 135. I feel too good and full of energy. My No# is 9460176480. I am very thankful to you. You have changed my life.

Ravi Kant Prasad
Q.No. NT/III/22

Narcotics Staff Colony Kota Raj.

Date: 17/11/10

Miss Pooja

My daughter Pooja age 20 years suffers from Lupus Nephritis. It is a serious Autoimmune disease. Doctors usually prescribe corticosteroids in this disease. I know the side effects of Steroids, so wanted to avoid these medicines. So I did some research on google.com and there I got telephone No# of Dr. O.P.Verma. I talked to him about Poona's problem. He prescribed 2-3 tbsp flaxseed oil daily along with some flaxseeds. He told us to blend oil with cottage cheese with hand blender nicely. I started this treatment on January, 2010 and stopped Steroids and other medicines prescribed by her doctor.

Pooja got lot of relief. Her doctors are also surprised that their treatment is very effective. Although I only know that she is not taking any of their medication. Wow! I am thankful to Dr. O.P.Verma

Manorama, Delhi

Anita Sahai

W/O Shailendra Nath Sahai Age 44 Years

My Husband suffers from Multiple Sclerosis since a few years. He is unable to walk or do any job. Treatment was not doing any good. Then I consulted Dr. O.P.Verma. He suggested to consume flaxseeds and cold-pressed flax oil.

Since 6 months he is continuously taking flaxseeds and oil. It looks as if somebody has done a miracle. My husband is has improved a lot.

My Publications

Cancer - Cause and Cure: Based on Quantum Physics developed by Dr. Johanna Budwig

http://www.amazon.com/Cancer-Quantum-Physics-developed-Johanna-ebook/dp/B00P3Y7BYG

Book Description

Publication Date: **October 31, 2014** | Age Level: **10 - 18** | Grade Level: **7 - 12**

***** A must have book for every cancer patient *****

This book provides an introduction of Dr. Budwig's cancer research and treatment. Johanna Budwig (1908-2003) was nominated for the Nobel Prize seven times. She was one of Germany's leading scientists of the 20th Century, a biochemist and cancer specialist with a special interest in essential fats.

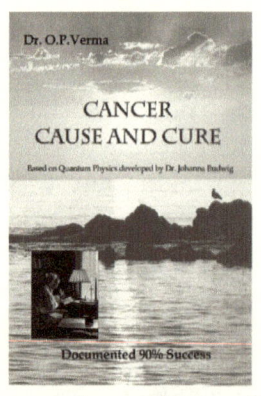

Otto Warburg proved that prime cause of cancer oxygen-deficiency in the cells. In absence of oxygen cells ferment glucose to produce energy, lactic acid is formed as a byproduct of fermentation. He postulated that sulfur containing protein and some unknown fat is required to attract oxygen in the cell.

In 1951 Dr. Budwig developed Paper Chromatography to identify fats. With this technique she proved that electron rich highly unsaturated Linoleic and Linolenic fatty acids were the undiscovered mysterious decisive fats in respiratory enzyme function that Otto Warburg had been unable to find. She studied the electromagnetic function of pi-electrons of the linolenic acid in the membranes of the microstructure of protoplasm, for all nerve function, secretions, mitosis, as well as cell break-down. This immediately caused lot of excitement in the scientific community. New doors could open in Cancer research.

Hydrogenated fats, including all Tran's fatty acids were proved as respiratory poisons.

Then Budwig decided to have human trials and gave flaxseed oil and quark to cancer patients. After three months, the patients began to improve in health and strength, the yellow green substance in their blood began to disappear, tumors gradually receded and at the same time the nutrients began to rise. This way Dr. Budwig had found a cure for cancer. It was a great victory and first milestone in the battle against cancer. Her treatment protocol is based on the consumption of flax seed oil with low fat cottage cheese, raw organic diet, mild exercise, and the healing powers of the sun. She treated approx. 2500 cancer patients during a 50 year period with this protocol till her death with over 90% documented success.

She was nominated 7 times for Nobel Prize but with a condition that she will use chemotherapy and radiotherapy with her protocol. They did not want to collapse the 200 billion dollar business over night. She always refused to support the damaging chemo and radio for the sake of humanity.

Lothar Hirneise is founder and President of People Against Cancer, Germany. He travels a lot in search of finding most successful alternative cancer therapies. He has been student of Dr. Johanna Budwig. He is a great researcher and writer on alternative healing. He is successfully treating thousands of cancer patients at his 3-E center in Germany. In the last few years he has interviewed several hundred final stage so-called survivors, meaning patients who were in the final stage of cancer and who are all healthy again today. Based on his findings he proposed a 3 E Program – The Mnemonic of Cancer Treatment.

1) Eat well
2) Eliminate
3) Energy

He noticed that 100% of all survivors, did the energy work. In approximately - say 80% of all patients, had changed their diet. And in at least 60% of all patients, took intensive detoxification rituals. This is the basis of his, so much talked about 3E Program for healing cancer.

Lothar Hirneise strongly supports holistic and spiritual approach and includes Visualization, Tumor Contract, Meditation, mild Yoga, Emotional Freedom Technique, Dr. Ryke Geerd Hamer's New German Medicine (Connection of unresolved stress and cancer), Detoxification techniques (Soda Bicarb bath, Epsom bath, Sauna, Colon Hydrotherapy, Coffee Enema etc.) in his 3 E Program.

The book also, describes about rare and miraculous herbs used in the treatment of Cancer like Turmeric, Black seed, Ginger, Mistle Toe, Aloe vera, , Echinecea, Lobelia, Essiac Tea, Pau d'arco Tea, Dandelion, Milk Thistle

Secrets of Success: Smart way to success for every student [Kindle Edition]

Book Description

Secrets of Success

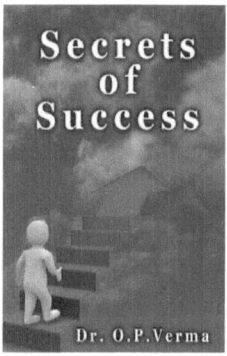

Normally people think that memory, intelligence or learning ability is a God gift and it is not possible to further improve or increase the brain powers. We take it for granted that it will remain as it is gifted to us by God. But the truth is just opposite. Understand that as you go to gym for workout to develop your six pack abs, feed your body with muscle building food and get sharp sculpted body shape. Friends, believe me if muscle can be built and remodeled, then why not your brain's hardware and circuit boards. If you feed your brain with proper food it needs, follow simple instructions and take advantage of neurobics or mnemonics, you can immensely increase your brain's abilities.

We have tremendous powers locked inside our brains, but we are not using them to full extent. Dr. William James, considered the father of modern psychology, pointed out that "the average human being uses only 10 percent of his mental capacity." We still have to find out how much power or secrets are hidden in our brain.

Nowadays scientists have discovered mysterious techniques and nutrients to boost our brain powers. Today I shall raise curtains from all these secrets; I shall disclose all hidden tricks and tips. Today you are going to learn how your CPU, the brain tightly packed in a bony cabinet, functions. I teach you how each component and microprocessors works and how the best insulation material can be prepared. I also disclose the right technique to sharpen your brain and to make you an intelligent and successful scholar.

Today you will learn how to crack every examination you face, solve every question, defeat every opponent and get highest possible marks. You are going to write new equation of education and success.

Friends, new boundaries and horizon of success is ready to welcome you. Today we shall discuss in detail about some great nutrients and supplements to boost your memory, learning, imagination, creativity and concentration. If you follow our suggestions and apply simple tricks you achieve a successful personality. This short e-book is going to prove a turning point in your life. Wish you luck. Visit us at http://memboy.blogspot.in

Bibliography

MNT Knowledge Center.com [Online]. - http://www.medicalnewstoday.com/articles/265990.php.
Nobelprize.org [Online]. - http://www.nobelprize.org/nobel_prizes/medicine/laureates/1931/ warb urg-bio.html. University of Maryland Medical Center [Online]. - http://umm.edu/health/medical/altmed/supplement/fiber.
About Health [Online]. - http://lowcarbdiets.about.com/od/nutrition/a/fiberbenefits.htm.
Omega-3 Fatty Acids [Online]. - http://themedicalbiochemistrypage.org/omegafats.php.
American Nutrition Association [Online]. - 1972. - http://americannutritionassociation.org/newsletter/flaxseed-neglectedfood.
Ben Green Field Fitness [Online]. - http://www.bengreenfieldfitness.com/2014/06/bulletproof-

coffeeenema/. Botanical.com [Online]. -
http://www.botanical.com/botanical/mgmh/b/burdoc87.html.
Botanicals.com [Online]. -
http://www.botanical.com/botanical/mgmh/l/lobeli38.html.
Botanicals.com [Online]. -
http://www.botanical.com/botanical/mgmh/m/mistle40.html.
Dr. Johanna Budwig Cancer The Problem And The Solution
[Book]. Dr. Johanna Budwig FlaxOil As A True Aid Against
Arthritis, Heart Infarction, Cancer, And Other Diseases [Book].
Dr. Johanna Budwig The Oil-Protein Diet Cookbook [Book]. -
Vancouver, Canada : Apple Publishing Co. Ltd., 1994. Cairns
George Cancer Tutor.com [Online]. -
http://www.cancertutor.com/dandelionroot/. Caisse Rene Rene
Caisse Tea [Online]. - http://renecaissetea.com/. Flax Council of
Canada Online]. -
http://www.flaxcouncil.ca/english/pdf/FlxPrmr_4ed_Chpt2.pdf.
Craig Gary The EFT Manual Paperback [Book]. - March 15,
2011 CureZone.com CureZone.com [Online]. -
http://curezone.com/forums/am.asp?i=67355. Doctor NDTV
[Online]. -
http://doctor.ndtv.com/faq/ndtv/fid/20230/Are_flax_seeds_benefi
cial_f or_osteoarthritis_patients.html. Dr Robert E. Willner M.D.
Ph.D. THE CANCER SOLUTION [Book]. - 1993. Ellie's Whole
Grains [Online]. - http://www.ellies-
wholegrains.com/lignan.html#axzz3NUEFVCsm. Elli's Whole
Grains [Online]. - http://www.ellies-wholegrains.com/flax-
mucilage.html. Udo Erasmas Fats That Heal, Fats That Kill
[Book]. - 1993. - p. www.udoerasmus.com/. Escher Ursula
BudwigDVDs.com [Online]. -
http://www.budwigdvds.com/articles/budwig-diet-protocol-
videos.htm. Essiac Facts.com [Online]. -
http://www.healthfreedom.info/turkey%20rhubarb%20v.%20indi
an%2 0rhubarb.htm. Essiac Facts.com [Online]. -
http://www.healthfreedom.info/sheep_sorrel.htm. Essiac
Facts.com [Online]. - http://essiacfacts.com/essiac-tea-
fordiabetes/. Euler Lee Cancer Defeated.com [Online]. -
http://www.cancerdefeated.com/newsletters/Plant-that-

CuresPractically-Everything.html. Feast without fear.com [Online]. - https://feastwithoutfear.wordpress.com/2012/12/01/understanding omega-3-and-omega-6-pathways-how-it-could-change-your-life/. Flax Awareness Society [Online]. - http://flaxindia.blogspot.in/2011/10/blog-post_247.html. Flax Awareness Society [Online]. - http://flaxindia.blogspot.in/2011/08/blog-post_9478.html. Flax Awareness Society [Online]. - http://flaxindia.blogspot.in/2011/08/blog-post_9478.html. Flax Awareness Society [Online]. - http://flaxindia.blogspot.in/2011/08/blog-post_3583.html. Flax Council of Canada [Online]. - http://www.flaxcouncil.ca/english/pdf/FF_Arrhythmia_R.pdf. Flax Council of Canada [Online]. - http://www.flaxcouncil.ca/english/pdf/FF_Immune_R4.pdf. Flax Council of Canada [Online]. - http://www.flax.com/lib/content/default/articles/2f68e876a73e54 d52d4 e7ef2cbeaeaf7/Flax%20-%20Inflammation.pdf. Flax Facts [Online]. - http://www.healthyflax.com/pdfs/FC_FlaxFactSheets_SportNutri tion.p df. Flaxseed MD [Online]. - http://www.flaxseedmd.com/flax-seedoil-articles-nutritional-superstar.asp. Grains Ellies Whole [Online]. - http://www.ellies-wholegrains.com/flax-seed-and-cholesterol.html#axzz3NUEFVCsm. Hamer Dr. Ryke Geerd CANCER, DISEASE OF THE PSYCHE [Book]. Health Freedom.com [Online]. - http://www.healthfreedom.info/sheep_sorrel.htm. Herb Wisdom.com [Online]. - http://www.herbwisdom.com/herbaloe-vera.html. Lothar Hirneise Chemotherapy Heals Cancer And World Is Flat [Book]. - [s.l.] : www.nexus-health.com, 2005. - Vol. 1. ICRF Independent Cancer Research Foundation Inc. Lee's Summit, Missouri. Cancer Tutor.com [Online]. - http://www.cancertutor.com/black_cumin/. Lignans for Life [Online]. - http://www.lignans.net/. Lignans for Life [Online]. - http://www.lignans.net/. Live Strong.com [Online]. -

158

http://www.livestrong.com/article/84062-flaxseed-benefits-skin/. Live Strong.com [Online]. -
http://www.livestrong.com/article/309033-the-keratin-skin-diet/. Love to Kow [Online]. -
http://vitamins.lovetoknow.com/Vitamin_for_Good_Hair_and_S kin. Minarsich Mike Bionatures [Online]. -
http://bionaturesblog.com/. Minarsich Mike http://budwigflax.blogspot.in/ [Online] // BioNatures Blog. -
http://budwigflax.blogspot.in/. Morris Diane H. Flax Council of Canada [Online]. -
http://www.flaxcouncil.ca/files/web/2008_Sept_aflaxlignan.pdf. MRGinseng.com [Online]. - http://en.mr-ginseng.com/turmeric/. Olson Sandra Budwig Videos.com [Online]. -
http://www.budwig-videos.com/categories/20071009_3. Osburn Lynn Seeds of Longevity and a New Golden Age [Online]. -
http://alchemylab.com/seeds_of_a_new_gold.htm. Paradise Vegetarial in [Online]. -
http://www.vegparadise.com/highestperch53.html. Philip E.Bizel M.D. Alive and Well [Online]. Power Your Diet.com [Online]. -
http://www.nutrition-andyou.com/dandelion-herb.html. PR Web [Online]. -
http://www.prweb.com/releases/AIDS/2007/prweb572849.htm. Puna Wai Ora Mind-Body Cancer Clinic [Online]. - 2006-2014 . - http://www.alternative-cancer-care.com/dr-ryke-geerd-hamer.html. Ragner Alex Brainy Weight Loss [Online]. -
http://www.brainyweightloss.com/flaxseed-health-benefits.html. S.A.Wilsons.com [Online]. -
http://www.sawilsons.com/coffee.htm. Schmid Ulla Healing Cancer Naturally [Online]. -
http://www.healingcancernaturally.com/budwigcompatiblepainm anage ment.html. Schmid Ulla Healing Cancer Naturally [Online]. -
http://www.healingcancernaturally.com/warburgcancer-causeprevention.html. SFGate [Online]. -
http://healthyeating.sfgate.com/benefitsflaxseed-lignans-8277.html. Sharma Pundit Vaibhav Nath [Online]. -
http://astrologervaibhava.blogspot.in/2010/12/blog-

post_7281.html. Skelton Clare The Budwig Diet / Protocol [Online]. - http://www.budwig-diet.co.uk/eldi-oils/. University of Maryland Medical Center [Online]. - http://umm.edu/health/medical/altmed/herb/echinacea. University of Maryland Medical Center [Online]. - http://umm.edu/health/medical/altmed/herb/stinging-nettle. Viviscal [Online]. - http://www.viviscal.com/blog/best-hairgrowth-vitamin-fuller-hair/. Voice Islamin [Online]. - http://www.islamicvoice.com/august.99/tibb.htm. Weil Dr. andrew [Online]. - http://www.drweil.com/drw/u/ART00662/osteoarthritis-treatment.html. Wellness Natural Liver Support.com [Online]. - http://www.liversupport.com/milkthistle.htm. WHFoods [Online]. - http://www.whfoods.com/genpage.php?tname=disease&dbid=3.

Index

5

5 alpha-reductase, 34

A

ADHD, 16, 73, 74, 75
AIDS, 36, 146
Alpha Linolenic Acid, 1
Alpha-Linolenic Acid, 15, 56
Aponechium, 130
Apple Cider Vinaigrette, 140
Apple cider vinegar & honey, 113
Arachidonic Acid, 17
Arrhythmias, 54, 55
Atherosclerosis, 50, 51

B

Balsamic Vinaigrette, 141
benign prostatic hyperplasia (BPH),
    35
Bionatures, 7
Biotin, 129, 130
Bitter Melon, 65
Black Seed, 65
Boswellia Serrata, 114
Brazil nut, 87, 119
Budwig- Compatible Pain Therapies,
    112
Budwig Diet, 84
Budwig Diet & Protocol - In Brief, 117
Budwig Diet Juicing Routine, 110

C

cafestol palmitate, 100
calcifications, 145
carboxylic acid, 14
Cartilage, 131
Charlemagne, 2
Chemo and Radio, 93

Cherries, 112
Cholesterol, 43, 52, 61
Chondroitin, 133
Chronic Inflammation, 57, 60
Cinnamon, 65
Cis configuration, 17
Cobalt 60 isotopes, 78
Coffee Enema, 100
Cognitive Decline, 74
Colostrum, 64
Constipation, 42
Constituents of Dietary Fiber, 38
copper, 128
Crime Cutter, 73
Cuticle, 125
Cytokine, 48

D

Dandruff, 127
Dental Care, 92
diabetes, 23, 25, 31, 57, 58, 59, 60,
    61, 63, 64, 65
Dietary fiber, 38
Docosahexanoic acid DHA, 15
Dr. Danial Daves, 36
Dr. Jeffrey Benabio, 124
Dr. Johanna Budwig
    Who developed Cancer treatment,
    78
Dr. Johanna Budwig's Works in
    English, 80
Dr. Otto Warburg
    Discovered the prime cause of
    cancer, 77

E

Egg Substitution, 140
Eicosanoid, 48
Eicosapentaanoic acid EPA, 15
Eldi oil, 96

Enterodiol, 29, 31
enterolactone, 29, 30, 33, 37
epidermis, 122
Epsom bath, 103

F

Federal Institute for Fat Research,
   81
Follicle, 126, 128
food cravings, 42, 60
Freudenstadt, Germany, 81
Functions of omega-3, 16

G

Ginger, 110, 133, 134, 154
Glucosamine sulfate, 133
glutathione S-transferase, 100
Goddess Parvati, 10
Grant Roberts, 136, 137

H

Hair follicles, 123
Herbs & supplements, 113
Hilary Swank, 136
Hippocmpus, 69
Hippocrates, 2
hormone binding globulin (SHBG), 36
Hulda, 3

I

Immune System, 47
insoluble fiber, 6, 41, 42, 44, 45
Insoluble fiber, 40
Interleukin – 6, 48
Interleukin 1B, 48

J

Juicers, 111
Juicing for the Budwig Protocol, 109

K

Kahweol, 100
keloid, 124
Kenneth Setchell, 28
Keratin, 126
keratinocytes, 126
KOMBUCHA, 112

L

Lemon Vinaigrette, 140
leukotrines, 61
Lignans, 6, 28, 29, 30, 31, 32, 33, 34,
   35, 36, 47, 61, 124
Linoleic Acid LA, 17
Linseed Goddess, 9
Linum usitatissimum, 1
low glycemic food, 58
lunula, 129
lupus erythematosus, 31, 49

M

Magnesium, 5, 64, 103
Mahatma Gandhi, 3
manganese, 128
Maria Treben's herbs, 113
Masticating juicer, 111
Matrix, 125
mayo salad dressing, 90
Medium chain FA, 14
Melanin, 123, 127
Melanocyte, 127
Membrane Phospholipids, 47
Memory, 64, 67, 68, 69, 74, 75
Memory decay, 68
memory process, 67
Metabolism of ALA, 25
Mike Minarsich, 7
Million Dollar Baby, 136
mnemonics, 70, 155
Moksha, 9
Mucilage, 42

N

Nail, 129
Neelpushpi, 9
neurotransmitters, 70, 74
Nigella Sativa, 65
NONI JUICE, 113

O

Oil Enema, 97
Oil Packs, 97
Oil-Protein Muesli, 85, 118
    Recipe, 86, 118
Oleolox – Budwig butter, 105
Omega-3, 21, 23, 24, 25, 40, 55, 58,
    60, 61, 70, 72, 73, 74, 123, 124,
    127, 130, 138, 140
Omega-6 / Omega-3 Metabolic
    Pathways, 21
Oregano Oil, 114
Osteoarthritis, 131, 132, 149

P

Paper Chromatography, 78
papilla, 125
Platelet- activating Factor, 48
Precautions of Budwig Diet, 92
Prohibitions of Budwig Protocol, 94,
    120
Prostaglandins, 19
Prostaglandins - Functions, 20
Protein, 5, 7, 59, 80, 90, 106, 112,
    127, 130, 135

R

Rebounder, 106
refined oil, 62
road to aging, disease & death, 23

S

Salad Platter, 89
Sauerkraut juice, 84

Science of Memory, 67
SDG, 28, 29, 30, 31, 33, 35
Sebaceous glands, 123
Sebum, 126
selenium, 24, 128
Short chain FA, 14
short-chain fatty acids, 45
Silica, 128
Sim Card of Mind, 74
Skin, 122, 123, 124
Soda bicarb bath, 104
Sodium bicarbonate as pain reliever,
    115
Soluble fiber, 6, 39, 44, 59
Sprouting flaxseeds, 142
Sun Therapy, 105
synovium, 131

T

The Colon World, 45
thermogenesis, 137
Thromboxane, 48
Trans configuration, 18
Trans Fats, 18
Transition Diet, 83
triglycerides, 16, 25, 52, 61, 65, 126
Tumor necrosis factor, 48
Turmeric, 114, 133, 154

U

Ulcerative Colitis, 43
Ultra wellness & longevity, 23

V

Vanadium, 65
Vitamin A, 127
Vitamin B Complex, 127
Vitamin C, 5, 128
Vitamin E, 5, 31, 128
vitamin H, 129

W

William Fischer, 7

Y

Yoga Nidra, 109

Z

Zero Carb food, 59
Zinc, 5, 128, 130